Neuro-Ophthalmology

REVIEW MANUAL

SIXTH EDITION

Lanning B. Kline, MD

EyeSight Foundation of Alabama Chair
Professor and Chairman
Department of Ophthalmology
University of Alabama School of Medicine
Birmingham, Alabama

Frank J. Bajandas, MD

Deceased

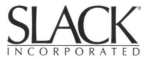

SLACK
INCORPORATED

Delivering the best in health care information and education worldwide www.slackbooks.com

ISBN: 978-1-55642-789-3

The procedures and practices described in this book should be implemented in a manner consistent with the professional standards set for the circumstances that apply in each specific situation. Every effort has been made to confirm the accuracy of the information presented and to correctly relate generally accepted practices. The authors, editor, and publisher cannot accept responsibility for errors or exclusions or for the outcome of the material presented herein. There is no expressed or implied warranty of this book or information imparted by it. Care has been taken to ensure that drug selection and dosages are in accordance with currently accepted/recommended practice. Due to continuing research, changes in government policy and regulations, and various effects of drug reactions and interactions, it is recommended that the reader carefully review all materials and literature provided for each drug, especially those that are new or not frequently used. Any review or mention of specific companies or products is not intended as an endorsement by the author or publisher.

SLACK Incorporated uses a review process to evaluate submitted material. Prior to publication, educators or clinicians provide important feedback on the content that we publish. We welcome feedback on this work.

Published by: SLACK Incorporated
                  6900 Grove Road
                  Thorofare, NJ 08086 USA
                  Telephone: 856-848-1000
                  Fax: 856-853-5991
                  www.slackbooks.com

Contact SLACK Incorporated for more information about other books in this field or about the availability of our books from distributors outside the United States.

Library of Congress Cataloging-in-Publication Data

Kline, Lanning B.
  Neuro-ophthalmology review manual / Lanning B. Kline, Frank J. Bajandas. -- 6th ed.
      p. ; cm.
  Includes bibliographical references and index.
  ISBN 978-1-55642-789-3 (alk. paper)
  1. Neuroophthalmology--Examinations, questions, etc. I. Bajandas, Frank J. II. Title.
  [DNLM: 1. Eye Diseases--Handbooks. 2. Eye--innervation--Handbooks. 3. Eye Manifestations--Handbooks. 4. Neurologic Manifestations--Handbooks. WW 39 K65n 2007]

RE725.K55 2007
617.7--dc22
                              2007024815

Printed in the United States of America.

Last digit is print number: 10   9   8   7   6   5   4   3   2   1

DEDICATION

Gentler the Path with Familiar Footsteps to Follow

This manual is dedicated to
Robert B. Daroff, MD
Joel S. Glaser, MD
J. Lawton Smith, MD

CONTENTS

Color Chart

ABOUT THE AUTHOR

Lanning B. Kline, MD, is a native of Edmonton, Alberta, Canada. He received his Bachelor of Arts degree from the University of Alberta and graduated from Duke University School of Medicine. He served an internship at Duke University Department of Medicine and a residency in the Department of Ophthalmology, McGill University, Montreal, Quebec, Canada. Dr. Kline completed fellowships in neuro-ophthalmology at the Montreal Neurological Institute and at the Bascom Palmer Eye Institute, Miami, Florida.

Dr. Kline has been a faculty member in the University of Alabama–Birmingham Department of Ophthalmology since 1979. In 1998 he became Professor and Chairman of the department, and in 2000 was appointed to the EyeSight Foundation of Alabama Endowed Chair in Ophthalmology.

Dr. Kline is certified by the American Board of Ophthalmology, is a member of the North American Neuro-Ophthalmology Society, and a Fellow of the American College of Surgeons. He recently celebrated his 30th wedding anniversary with his wife, Ricki. Their two children, Aaron and Evelyn, are both professionally employed in California.

CONTRIBUTING AUTHORS

John E. Carter, MD
Associate Professor of Neurology and Ophthalmology
University of Texas Health Science Center
San Antonio, Texas

Richard H. Fish, MD, FACS
Vitreoretinal Consultants
Clinical Associate Professor
Department of Ophthalmology
Baylor College of Medicine
Houston, Texas

Christopher A. Girkin, MD, MSPH, FACS
Professor and Director, Glaucoma Service
Department of Ophthalmology
University of Alabama School of Medicine
Birmingham, Alabama

Saunders L. Hupp, MD
Vision Partners, LLC
Clinical Professor of Ophthalmology
University of South Alabama
Mobile, Alabama

Angela R. Lewis, MD
Assistant Professor of Ophthalmology
Department of Ophthalmology
Tulane University School of Medicine
New Orleans, Louisiana

Patrick S. O'Connor, MD
Clinical Professor of Ophthalmology
University of Texas Health Science Center
San Antonio, Texas

Jennifer T. Scruggs, MD
Assistant Professor
Department of Ophthalmology
University of Alabama School of Medicine
Birmingham, Alabama

Mark F. Walker, MD
Associate Professor of Neurology
Case Western Reserve University and Veterans Affairs Medical Center
Cleveland, Ohio

Milton F. White, Jr, MD
Retina Consultants of Alabama
Clinical Associate Professor
Department of Ophthalmology
University of Alabama School of Medicine
Birmingham, Alabama

INTRODUCTION

In order to remain up-to-date, *Neuro-Ophthalmology Review Manual* must keep pace with the ever-increasing knowledge base of the subspecialty. Now in print for more than 25 years, this Sixth Edition remains focused on its primary objective: "A readable compendium of 'no-nonsense' neuro-ophthalmology."

I am particularly grateful to Mark F. Walker, MD, in the reorganization of Chapter 2 and revision of Chapter 3. Similarly, John E. Carter, MD, has rewritten Chapter 15, outlining those headache syndromes that are important in neuro-ophthalmic diagnosis, and Jennifer T. Scruggs, MD, has improved Chapter 14. Once again, all chapters have had references updated, and David Fisher has revised and improved a number of the illustrations throughout the text.

It has been almost three decades since Frank J. Bajandas, MD, conceived this "nuts-and-bolts" guide of neuro-ophthalmology. All the authors have been diligent in maintaining his clear and direct style in order to demystify but not oversimplify the core material of neuro-ophthalmology. His legacy continues and I hope he would be proud of our efforts.

—*LBK*

Chapter 1

Visual Fields

Lanning B. Kline, MD

I. **Traquair's definition of the visual field**

A. Island of vision in a sea of blindness (Figure 1-1). The peak of the island represents the point of highest acuity—the fovea—while the "bottomless pit" represents the blind spot—the optic disc

II. **For clinical testing, the visual field can be divided into two areas (Figure 1-2)**

A. Central: 30-degree radius

B. Peripheral: beyond 30 degrees

III. **Visual field testing**

A. Stimuli: testing the island of vision at various levels requires targets that vary in:
1. Size
2. Luminance
3. Color

B. Background luminance: at 31.5 asp (apostilb) the fovea has the highest sensitivity; able to detect dimmest and smallest targets

C. Field testing methods
1. Can be examined with Amsler grid, confrontation techniques, kinetic perimetry, automated perimetry
2. Amsler grid—useful in detecting subtle central and paracentral scotomas. When held at one third of a meter from the patient, each square subtends 1 degree of visual field
3. Confrontation techniques
    a. Quick screen for hemianopia and altitudinal defects
    b. Nonquantitative; requires practiced examiner
    c. See Chapter 20
4. Kinetic perimetry (Figure 1-3)
    a. Moving stimulus is used
    b. Both size and luminance of stimulus may be altered

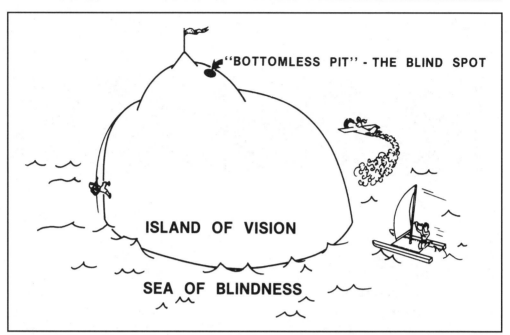

Figure 1-1. Traquair's definition of the visual field—island of vision in a sea of blindness.

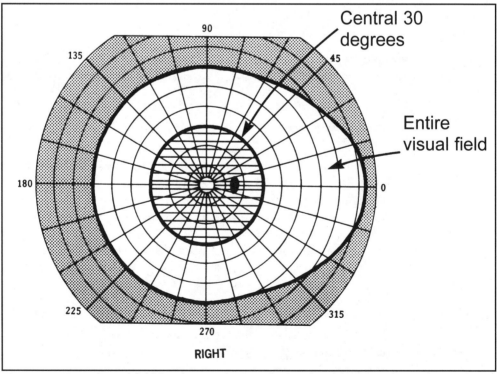

Figure 1-2. Central visual field (30-degree radius) can be tested with automated perimetry, while the entire visual field requires use of manual perimetry.

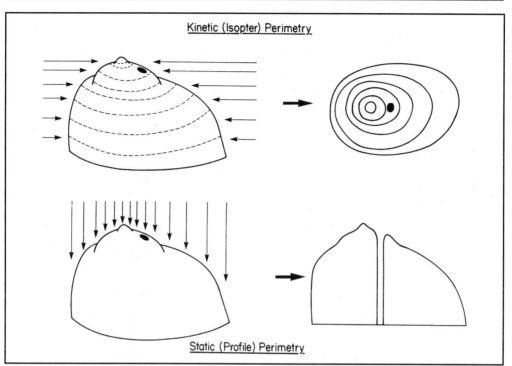

Kinetic (Isopter) Perimetry

Static (Profile) Perimetry

Figure 1-3. Kinetic perimetry: each set of target size-color-intensity and background illumination determines a different level of the island being tested and results in a different oval-shaped cross-section or isopter; note the six isopters at the right, the result of testing six levels of the island. Static perimetry: the target is held stationary at different points along the selected meridians; the intensity of the target is slowly increased until it is detected by the patient; the intensity required determines the upper level (the greatest sensitivity) of the island at this point.

    c.   Map the contours of the island of vision at different levels, resulting in one isopter for each level tested

    d.   Evaluation of the entire visual field

    e.   Particularly helpful in detecting:

        i.   Ring scotoma (retinitis pigmentosa)

        ii.   Nasal step (glaucoma)

        iii.   Temporal crescent (occipital lobe)

        iv.   Non-organic field lens—see Chapter 17

    f.   Disadvantages

        i.   Variable reproducibility

        ii.   Dependent on skill of perimetrist

        iii.   Perimetrist bias may affect results

5.   Static perimetry (see Figure 1-3)

    a.   Stimulus location fixed

    b.   Stimulus size standardized

    c.   Vary stimulus luminance to assess light sensitivity at various points in visual field

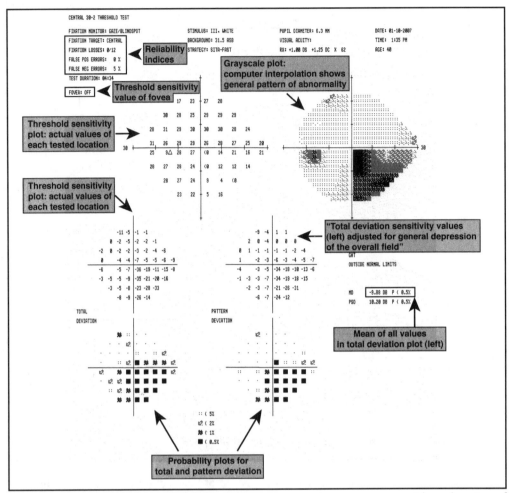

Figure 1-4. Printout of Humphrey 30-2 automated state perimetry program, with explanation of statistical analysis, grayscale, and probability plots.

        d.   Standard automated perimetry is now the most widely used form of perimetry (Figure 1-4)

        e.   Advantages include standardized test strategies, well-established normative database for comparison, careful monitoring of fixation behavior, computerized storage of all data

    6.   Factors affecting visual field testing

        a.   Testing conditions: background luminance, stimulus size, stimulus deviation, stimulus spectral composition

        b.   Physiologic: refractive error, pupil size, ptosis, media opacities

        c.   Attention: fatigue, practice/learning effects

        d.   Response errors: fixation instability, testing artifacts (eg, lens rim obstruction, misalignment)

IV.   Anatomy of the visual pathways (Figure 1-5)

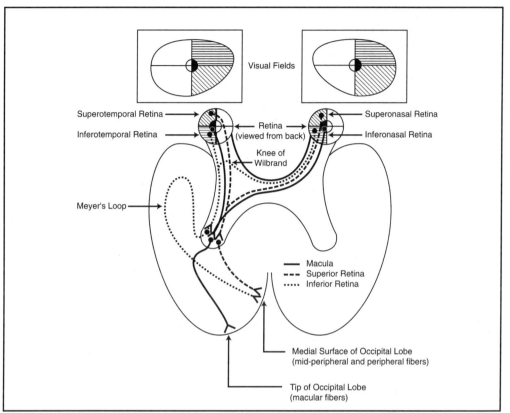

Figure 1-5. Anatomy of visual pathways.

A. The visual field and retina have an inverted and reversed relationship. Relative to the point of fixation, the upper visual field falls on the inferior retina (below the fovea), lower visual field on the superior retina, nasal visual field on the temporal retina, and temporal visual field on the nasal retina

B. Nasal fibers of ipsilateral eye cross in the chiasm join uncrossed temporal fibers of the contralateral eye → optic tract → synapse in lateral geniculate nucleus (LGN) → optic radiation → terminate in the visual cortex (area 17) of the occipital lobe

C. Inferonasal retinal fibers decussate in the chiasm and travel anteriorly in the contralateral optic nerve before passing into the optic tract. They form "Wilbrand's knee"

D. While the presence of Wilbrand's knee has been challenged (Horton, 1997), it still appears to have clinical relevance (Karanjia & Jacobson, 1999)

E. Lower retinal fibers and their projections lie in the lateral portion of the optic tract and ultimately terminate in the inferior striate cortex on the lower bank of the calcarine fissure. Upper retinal fibers project through the medial optic tract and ultimately terminate in the superior striate cortex

F. LGN. Visual information from ipsilateral eye synapses in layers 2, 3, 5; from contralateral in layers 1, 2, 6. Macular vision is subserved by the hilum, and peripheral field by the medial and lateral horns (Figure 1-15)

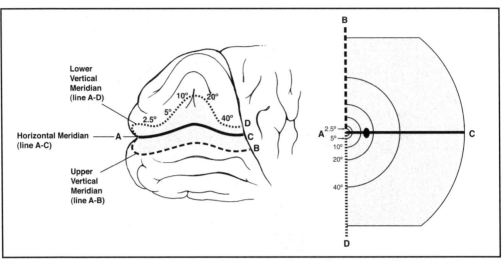

Figure 1-6. Medial view of the left occipital lobe with calcarine fissure opened, exposing the striate cortex. Dashed and solid lines represent coordinates of the visual field.

G. The central (30 degrees) visual field occupies a disproportionately large area (83%) of the visual cortex. The vertical hemianopic meridians are represented along the border of the calcarine lips, while the horizontal meridian follows the contour of the base of the calcarine fissure (Figure 1-6)

V. **Interpretation of visual field defects**

A. Ten key points to remember
1. Optic nerve-type field defects
2. "Rules of the road" for the optic chiasm
3. Optic tract—LGN defects
4. Superior-inferior separation in the temporal lobe
5. Superior-inferior separation in the parietal lobe
6. Central homonymous hemianopia
7. Macular sparing
8. Congruity
9. Optokinetic nystagmus (OKN)
10. Temporal crescents

B. Optic nerve-type field defects
1. Retinal nerve fibers enter the optic discs in a specific manner (Figure 1-7)
2. Nerve fiber bundle (NFB) defects are of the following three main types:
    a. Papillomacular bundle: macular fibers that enter the temporal aspect of the disc. A defect in this bundle of nerve fibers results in one of the following:
        i. Central scotoma (Figure 1-8): a defect covering central fixation
        ii. Centrocecal scotoma (see Figure 1-8): a central scotoma connected to the blind spot (cecum)
        iii. Paracentral scotoma (see Figure 1-8): a defect of some of the fibers of the papillomacular bundle lying next to, but not involving, central fixation

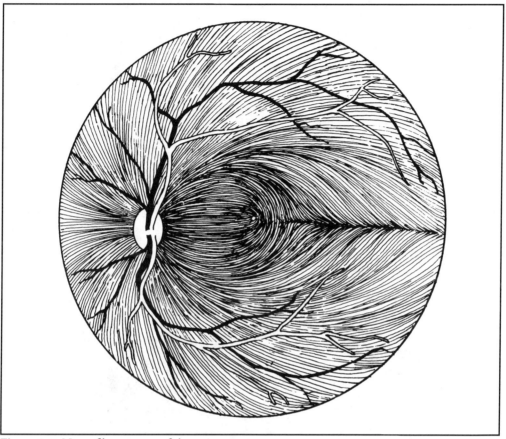

Figure 1-7. Nerve fiber pattern of the retina.

    b.   Arcuate NFB: fibers from the retina temporal to the disc enter the superior and inferior poles of the disc (see Figure 1-7). A defect of these bundles may cause one of the following:

        i.   Arcuate scotoma or defect (Figure 1-9): due to involvement of arcuate NFBs

        ii.   Seidel scotoma (see Figure 1-9): a defect in the proximal portion of the NFB, causing a comma-shaped extension of the blind spot

        iii.   Nasal step (see Figure 1-9): a defect in the distal portion of the arcuate NFB. Since the superior and inferior arcuate bundles do not cross the horizontal raphe of the temporal retina, a nasal step defect respects the horizontal (180 degree) meridian

        iv.   Isolated scotoma within arcuate area (see Figure 1-9): defect of the intermediate portion of the arcuate NFB

    c.   Nasal NFBs: fibers that enter the nasal aspect of the disc course in a straight (nonarcuate) fashion. The defect in this bundle results in a wedge-shaped temporal scotoma arising from the blind spot and does not necessarily respect the temporal horizontal meridian (see Figure 1-9)

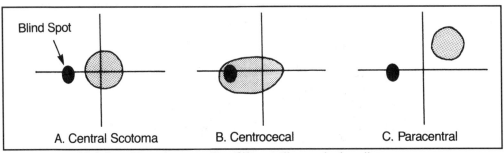

Figure 1-8. Field defects due to interruption of the papillomacular bundle.

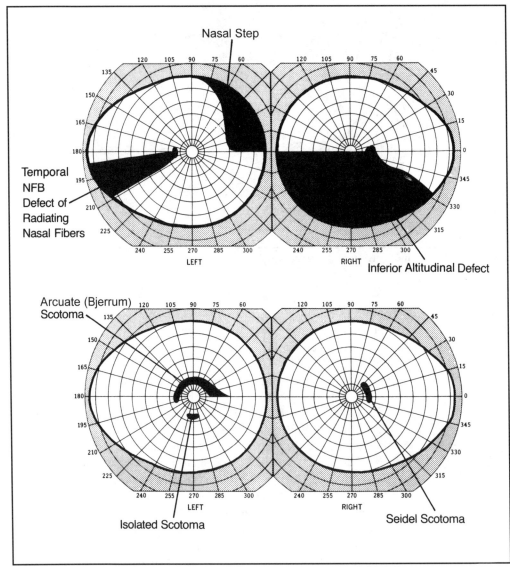

Figure 1-9. Composite diagram depicting different optic nerve-type field defects.

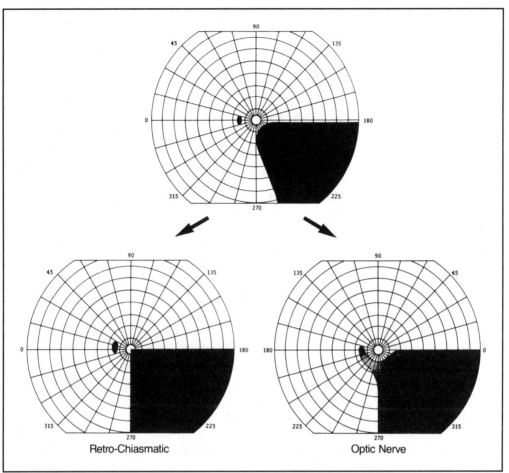

Figure 1-10. The key question in a patient with a quadrantic visual field defect: does the field defect go to fixation (retrochiasmatic lesion) or to the blind spot (optic nerve lesion)?

3. Lesions at or behind the chiasm tend to cause hemianopic field defects originating from the point of fixation and respecting the vertical meridian

4. Optic nerve lesions cause field defects corresponding to one of the three major NFB defects described above. NFB defects originate from the blind spot, not from the fixation point, and do not respect the vertical meridian, but do respect the nasal horizontal meridian

5. The key question, therefore, in a patient with a quadrantic field defect is: does the field defect go to fixation or to the blind spot (Figure 1-10)?

6. Additional clinical findings supporting the diagnosis of optic neuropathy as the cause of the field defect include:

    a. Decreased visual acuity: patients with isolated retrochiasmatic lesions do not have decreased visual acuity unless the lesions are bilateral, then the visual acuities will be equal; if a patient has hemianopic field defects with unequal visual acuities, then look for a lesion around the chiasm (affecting the optic nerves asymmetrically)

      b.   Patients with decreased (or suspected decreased) visual acuity can be further tested with:

         i.   Light-brightness comparison (eye with optic neuropathy will see the light as "less bright")

         ii.   Color perception comparison (color plates or Mydriacyl [Alcon Laboratories, Fort Worth, Tex] bottle cap) (eye with optic neuropathy will have diminished color perception)

         iii.   Light-stress recovery time (eye with maculopathy will have delayed recovery visual acuity after bleaching with light)

         iv.   Afferent pupillary defect test ("swinging flashlight" or Marcus Gunn test—see Chapter 8)

         v.   Tests i through iv may help in distinguishing cases of decreased visual acuity due to macular disease from those due to optic nerve disease

         vi.   Visual-evoked potentials (VEPs)

         vii.   Ophthalmoscopic evidence of optic disc abnormality (eg, pallor, cupping, drusen)

    7.   Rarely, optic nerve disease (compression, demyelination) may cause a monocular temporal hemianopia (relative afferent pupillary defect [RAPD] present as well). Lesion is posterior enough to disrupt ipsilateral crossing nasal fibers but too anterior to affect contralateral ones. Must distinguish from functional visual field loss (see Chapter 17, IV, A)

C.   "Rules of the road" for the optic chiasm:

    1.   Three rules describe the course of major fiber bundles in the chiasm:

      a.   The nasal retinal fibers (including the nasal half of the macula) of each eye cross in the chiasm to the contralateral optic tract. Temporal fibers remain uncrossed. Thus, a chiasmal lesion will cause a bitemporal hemianopia due to interruption of decussating nasal fibers (Figure 1-11)

      b.   Lower retinal fibers project through the optic nerve and chiasm to lie laterally in the tracts; upper retinal fibers will lie medially (there is a 90-degree rotation of fibers from the nerves through the chiasm into the tracts)

      c.   Inferonasal retinal fibers cross into the chiasm and cross anteriorly approximately 4 mm in the contralateral optic nerve (Wilbrand's knee) before turning back to join uncrossed inferotemporal temporal fibers in the optic tract (junctional scotoma). Existence of Wilbrand's knee is controversial (see Chapter 1, IV, D)

    2.   "Macular" crossing fibers are distributed throughout the chiasm and if primarily affected, cause a "central" bitemporal hemianopia (Figure 1-12)

    3.   Clinical "pearl": if a patient comes in with poor vision in the left eye, the important eye for visual examination is the right due to involvement of Wilbrand's knee. The lesion is now intracranial at the junction of the left optic nerve and chiasm. The field defects constitute a junctional scotoma (Figure 1-13)

D.   Optic tract—LGN defects

    1.   All retrochiasmatic lesions result in a contralateral homonymous hemianopia

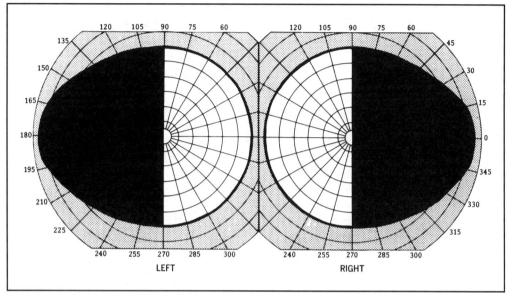

Figure 1-11. Bitemporal hemianopia due to interruption of decussating nasal fibers in the chiasm.

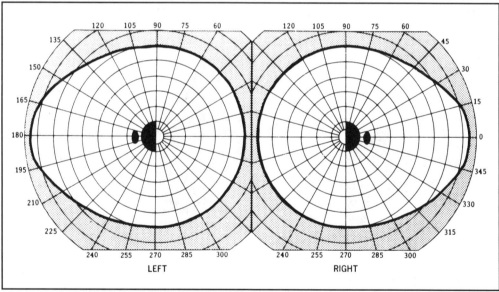

Figure 1-12. A chiasmatic lesion may affect only the decussating nasal-macular fibers, resulting in a central bitemporal hemianopia. Therefore, a complete visual field evaluation of a patient suspected of a chiasmatic lesion must include examination of the central field.

2. Congruity describes incomplete homonymous hemianopic defects that are identical in all attributes: location, shape, size, depth, slope of margins

3. **Remember:** the more posterior (toward the occipital cortex) the lesion in the postchiasmal visual pathways, the more likely the defects will be congruous

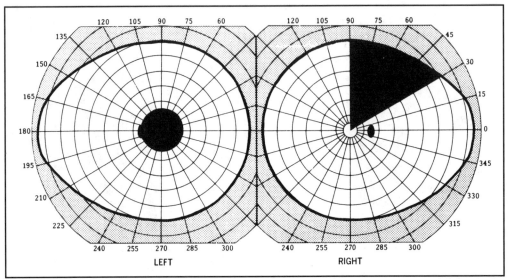

Figure 1-13. Junctional scotoma: a central scotoma in one eye with a superior-temporal defect in the fellow eye; indicates a lesion at the junction of the optic nerve (left eye in this case) and the chiasm.

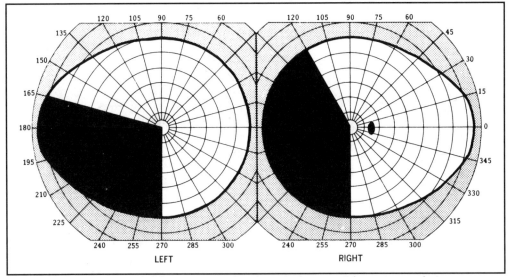

Figure 1-14. Incongruous left homonymous hemianopia due to a right optic tract lesion.

4.   In the optic tracts and LGN, nerve fibers of corresponding points (retinal positions of the two eyes that image the same position in visual space) do not yet lie adjacent to one another. This leads to incongruous visual field defects (Figure 1-14)

5.   In the LGN, afferent fibers are organized into alternating layers; crossed fibers terminate in layers 1, 4, 6 and uncrossed in 2, 3, 5

6.   Criteria for optic tract syndrome

   a.   Incongruous homonymous hemianopia

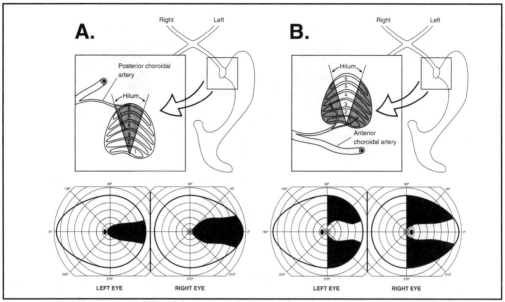

Figure 1-15. (A) Posterior choroidal artery occlusion leads to homonymous horizontal sectoranopia. (B) Anterior choroidal artery occlusion causes sector-sparing homonymous hemianopia.

    b.   Bilateral retinal nerve fiber layer atrophy or optic (occasionally "bow-tie") atrophy (see Chapter 10, III, G and Figure 10-2)

    c.   Pupillary abnormalities

        i.   RAPD: on side opposite the lesion (eye with temporal field loss)

        ii.   Wernicke's pupil: light stimulation of a "blind" retina causes no pupillary reaction, while light projected on an "intact" retina produces normal pupillary constriction

        iii.   Behr's pupil: anisocoria with larger pupil on the side of hemianopia; probably does not exist

    7.   LGN field defect

        a.   Visual information from ipsilateral eye synapses in layers 2, 3, 5; from contralateral in layers 1, 2, 6. Macular vision is subserved by the hilum and peripheral field by the medial and lateral horns

        b.   Types of defects:

            i.   Incongruous homonymous hemianopia

            ii.   Unique sector and sector-sparing defects due to dual blood supply of LGN from anterior and posterior choroidal arteries (Figure 1-15)

E.   Superior-inferior separation in the temporal lobe

    1.   Inferior fibers (ipsilateral inferotemporal fibers and contralateral inferonasal fibers) course anteriorly from the lateral geniculate body into the temporal lobe, forming Meyer's loop approximately 2.5 cm (range 2.4 to 2.8 cm) from the anterior tip of the temporal lobe. They are anatomically separated from the superior retinal fibers, which course directly back in the optic radiations of the parietal lobe (see Figure 1-5)

    2.   Inferior "macular" fibers do not cross as far anteriorly in the temporal lobe

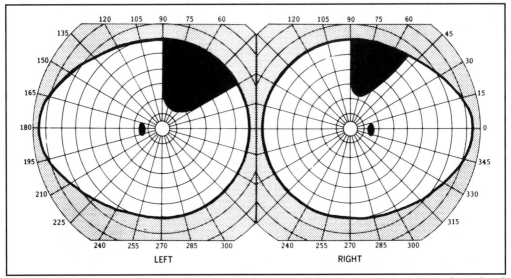

Figure 1-16. Anterior temporal lobe lesion of Meyer's loop produces incongruous, midperipheral and peripheral-contralateral, homonymous, superior ("pie in the sky") quadrantanopia. This is an example of a patient with a left temporal lobe lesion.

      3.   Anterior temporal lobe lesions tend to produce midperipheral and peripheral contralateral homonymous superior quadrantanopia ("pie in the sky" field defect) (Figure 1-16)

      4.   More extensive temporal lobe lesions may cause field defects that extend to the inferior quadrants, but hemianopia will be "denser" superiorly

  F. Superior-inferior separation in the parietal lobe

      1.   Superior fibers (ipsilateral superotemporal fibers and contralateral superonasal fibers) course directly through the parietal lobe to lie superiorly in the optic radiation

      2.   Inferior fibers course through the temporal lobe (Meyer's loop) and lie inferiorly in the optic radiation

      3.   Thus, there is "correction" of the 90-degree rotation of the visual fibers that occur through the chiasm into the tracts

      4.   Parietal lobe lesions tend to affect superior fibers first, resulting in contralateral inferior homonymous quadrantanopia (Figure 1-17) or a homonymous hemianopia "denser" inferiorly (Figure 1-18)

      5.   Two signs described with parietal lobe lesions:

          a.   Spasticity of conjugate gaze: tonic deviation of eyes to the side opposite a parietal lesion during an attempt to produce Bell's phenomenon (see Chapter 2)

          b.   OKN asymmetry: evoked nystagmus is dampened when stimuli are moved in the direction of the damaged parietal lobe (see Chapter 1, V, J)

  G. Central homonymous hemianopia

      1.   In the visual cortex, the macular representation is located on the tips of the occipital lobes

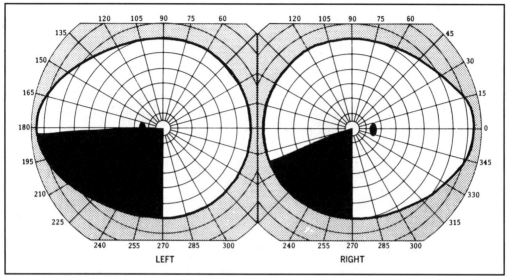

Figure 1-17. Parietal lobe lesions tend to affect the inferior, contralateral visual field quadrants first. This is an example of a patient with a right parietal lobe lesion.

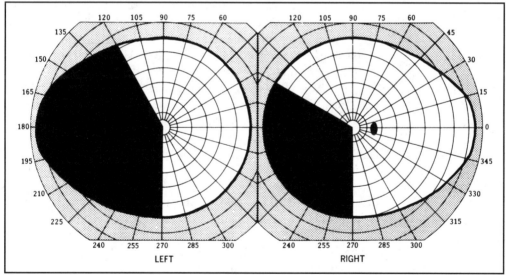

Figure 1-18. Incongruous left homonymous hemianopia.

    2.   The macular representation is separated from the cortical representation of the midperipheral and peripheral visual fields. These fibers terminate on the medial surface of the occipital lobes (see Figure 1-5)

    3.   A lesion affecting the tip of the occipital lobe tends to produce a central homonymous hemianopia (Figure 1-19)

H.   Macular sparing

    1.   The macular area of the visual cortex is a watershed area with respect to blood supply (Figure 1-20)

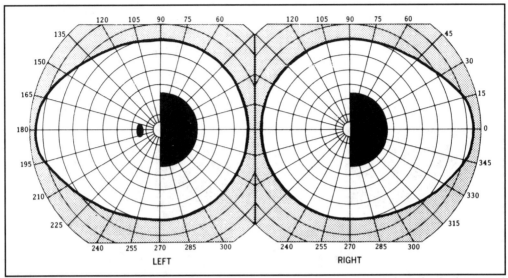

Figure 1-19. A lesion affecting only the tip of the occipital lobe produces a defect of only the central homonymous hemifields. This is an example of a patient with a left occipital tip lesion.

a.   The "macular" visual cortex is supplied by terminal branches of posterior and middle cerebral arteries

b.   The visual cortex subserving the midperipheral and peripheral field is supplied only by the posterior cerebral artery. The area is supplied by a more proximal (not a terminal) vessel

c.   Therefore, when there is obstruction of flow through the posterior cerebral artery, ipsilateral macular visual cortex may be spared because of blood supply provided by the terminal branches of the middle cerebral artery. This may be an explanation for "macular sparing"

d.   However, when there is a generalized hypoperfusion state (eg, intraoperative hypotension), the first area of the visual cortex to be affected is that supplied by terminal branches—the macular visual cortex—resulting in a central homonymous hemianopia (see Figure 1-19)

2.   In order to qualify as "macular sparing," at least 5 degrees of the macular field must be spared in both eyes on the side of the hemianopia (Figure 1-21)

3.   Macular sparing may at times be an artifact of testing. The patient may shift fixation, anticipating the appearance of the test object

4.   If a patient with a complete homonymous hemianopia is found to have sparing of the macula, then he or she is most likely to have an occipital lobe lesion; however, the majority of patients with occipital lobe lesions demonstrate a splitting of the macula (Figure 1-22); therefore, macular sparing is helpful only if present

5.   Bilateral homonymous hemianopias with macular sparing produce constricted visual fields (with normal fundi) (Figure 1-23). The differential diagnosis of constricted visual fields also includes:

a.   Non-organic visual field loss

b.   Glaucoma

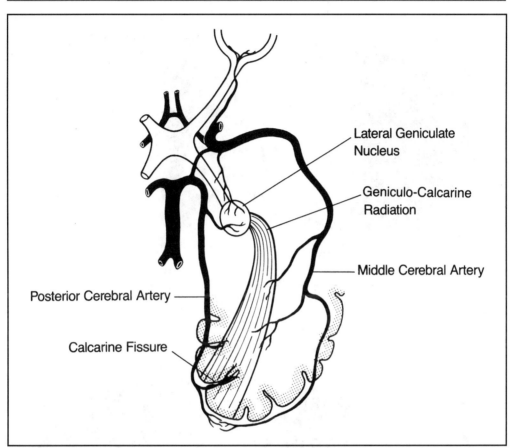

Figure 1-20. The tip of the occipital lobe, where the macular or central homonymous hemifields are represented, is supplied by terminal branches of the middle and posterior cerebral arteries; it is referred to as a watershed area. The medial surface of the occipital lobe is supplied by more proximal (not terminal) branches of the posterior cerebral artery.

        c.   Optic disc drusen

        d.   Post-papilledema optic atrophy

        e.   Retinitis pigmentosa

    6.   Items b through e listed above all have abnormal fundi and should be easily diagnosed. Differential from non-organic field loss requires fields done at 1 and 2 meters (Figure 1-24)

I.   Congruity

    1.   Homonymous hemianopic field defects are said to be congruous when the defect is not complete (ie, does not occupy the entire half of the field) and the defect extends to the same angular meridian in both eyes (Figure 1-25; the hemianopic defect extends to the 137-degree meridian in each eye)

    2.   Complete homonymous hemianopia (see Figure 1-22) cannot be categorized as "congruous" because it is complete

    3.   Figure 1-26 shows an example of incongruity: the hemianopia of the left eye extends to the 160-degree meridian while the hemianopia of the right eye extends to the 115-degree meridian

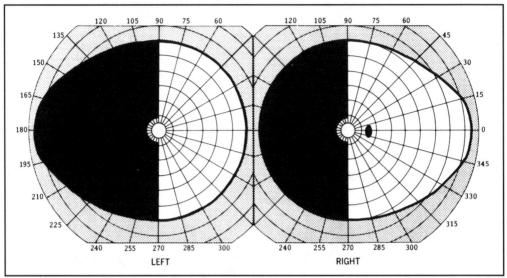

Figure 1-21. Left homonymous hemianopia with "sparing" of the left half of the macular field of each eye.

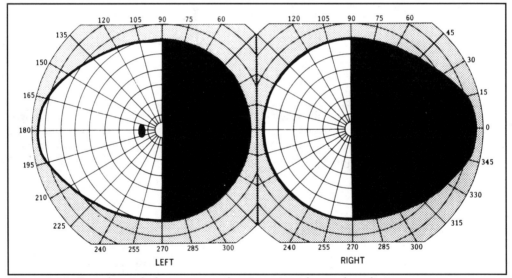

Figure 1-22. Complete right homonymous hemianopia with macular splitting.

4. Optic tract lesions tend to produce markedly incongruous field defects
5. The more congruous a homonymous hemianopia, the nearer the lesion will be to the occipital cortex (ie, more posterior in the visual pathways)
6. Congruity is due to the fact that a lesion affects nerve fibers from corresponding retinal points that lie adjacent to one another

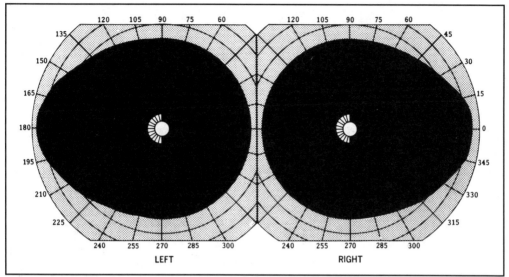

Figure 1-23. Bilateral homonymous hemianopias with macular sparing.

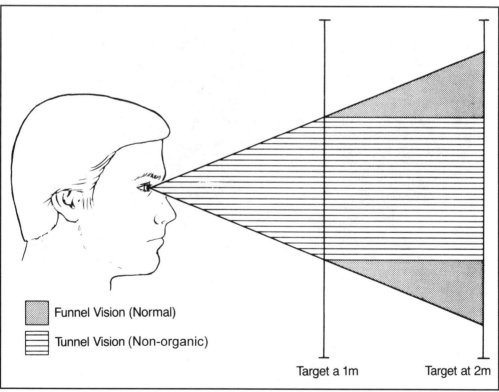

Figure 1-24. Visual fields performed at 1 and 2 meters.

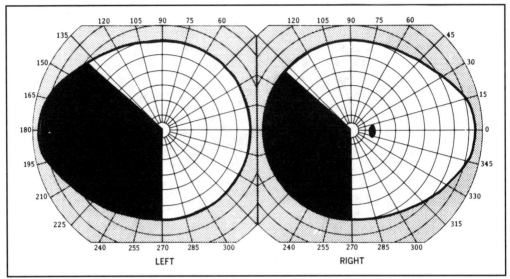

Figure 1-25. Congruous left homonymous hemianopia.

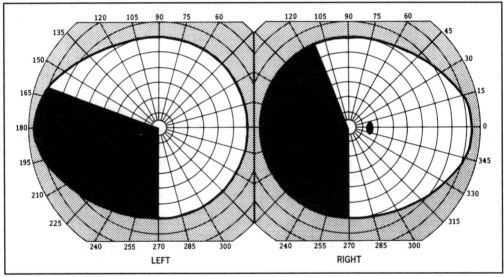

Figure 1-26. Incongruous left homonymous hemianopia.

J.   OKN

1.   The precise pathways of the optokinetic system are unknown in humans but may share pathways carrying smooth pursuit commands. This pathway extends from the visual association areas (18 and 19) to the horizontal gaze center in the pons (see Chapter 2)

2.   The pathway in the left visual association area will terminate in the left pontine gaze center, resulting in pursuit movement of the eyes to the left. Similarly, the pathway originating in the right cerebral hemisphere generates pursuit eye movements to the right

3. A patient with a purely occipital lobe lesion (even if resulting in a complete homonymous hemianopia) will have no difficulty with pursuit, since the pathways begin more anteriorly. OKN response will be symmetric

4. A patient with homonymous hemianopia due to a parietal lobe lesion will have deficient pursuit eye movements to the side of the lesion, resulting in asymmetric OKN. The OKN will be decreased when the drum is rotated toward the side of the lesion

5. Patients with homonymous hemianopia due to an optic tract, temporal lobe, or purely occipital lobe lesion will have symmetric OKN to both sides

6. Cogan's dictum
   a. Homonymous hemianopia + asymmetric OKN—probably parietal lobe lesion; most likely mass
   b. Homonymous hemianopia + symmetric OKN—probably occipital lobe lesion; most likely vascular infarction

K. Temporal crescents
1. When we fixate with both eyes and achieve fusion of the visual information gained by both eyes, there is superimposition of the corresponding portions of the visual fields: the central 60-degree radius of field in each eye

2. There remains, in each eye, a temporal crescent of field for which there are no corresponding visual points in the other eye (Figure 1-27)

3. This temporal crescent of field, perceived by a nasal crescent of retina, is represented in the contralateral visual cortex in the most anterior portion of the medial surface of the occipital lobe (along the calcarine fissure)

4. Representation of the temporal crescent occupies less than 10% of total surface area of striate cortex

5. If a patient is found to have a homonymous hemianopia with sparing of the temporal crescent (Figure 1-28), then he or she probably has an occipital lobe lesion since this is the only site where the temporal crescent of fibers are separated from the other nasal fibers of the contralateral eye

VI. **Special visual field cases**

A. Pseudobitemporal hemianopia
1. Field defects that do not respect the vertical meridian, but rather "slope" across it (Figure 1-29)
2. Causes include:
   a. Uncorrected refractive errors (myopia, astigmatism)
   b. Tilted optic discs
   c. Enlarged blind spots in papilledema
   d. Large central or centrocecal scotomas
   e. Sectoral retinitis pigmentosa (mainly in nasal quadrants)
   f. Overhanging eyelid tissue

B. Binasal hemianopia
1. Most nasal field defects are due to arcuate scotomas
2. Rarely, true unilateral or bilateral nasal hemianopia may occur with defects having no arcuate connection to the blind spot and, to some extent, respecting the vertical meridian

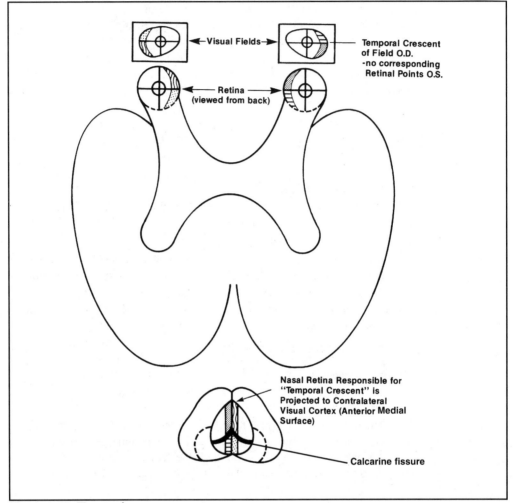

Figure 1-27. Temporal crescent.

3. Never as a result of chiasmal compression
4. May be due to pressure upon the temporal aspect of the optic nerve and the anterior angle of the chiasm or near the optic canal; in these locations, a lesion may affect only temporal retinal fibers. The fibers cannot be selectively obstructed in the lateral chiasm
5. Cause includes aneurysm, tumor (pituitary adenoma), vascular infarction

C. Monocular temporal hemianopia
1. Rare manifestation of visual pathway damage
2. May be seen with comprehensive lesion (pituitary tumor, meningioma, craniopharyngioma), optic disc anomaly (dysversion, optic nerve hypoplasia), or optic neuritis
3. In all cases a RAPD is present, with or without optic disc pallor
4. If RAPD absent, consider non-organic cause

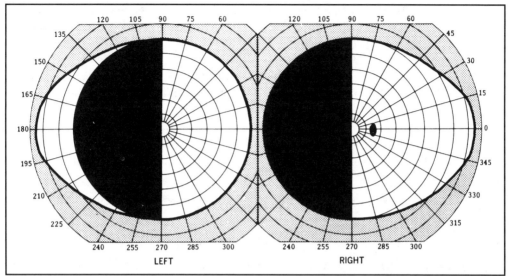

Figure 1-28. Left homonymous hemianopia with sparing of the temporal crescent of the left eye.

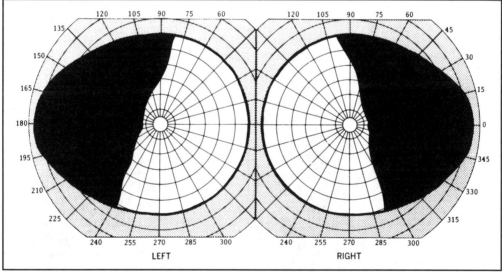

Figure 1-29. Pseudobitemporal hemianopia. Field defects do not respect the vertical meridian.

5. Attributed to involvement of ipsilateral optic nerve close enough to chiasm to impair crossing nasal fibers, but too anterior to affect crossing nasal retinal fibers from the contralateral eye

D. Big blind spot syndrome
   1. Sudden onset of temporal scotoma centered on the physiologic blind spot in one or both eyes
   2. Often accompanied by photopsia or scintillations in the blind spot
   3. Predilection for females

4. Associated with a variety of disorders including: some of the white dot syndromes (multiple evanescent white dot syndrome [MEWDS], multifocal choroiditis [MFC], acute zonal occult outer retinopathy [AZOOR], acute macular neuroretinopathy [AMN])

5. Optic disc may appear normal or mildly swollen

6. Full-field and multifocal electroretinography (ERG) abnormalities may be found

7. Etiology: transient peripapillary or diffuse photoreceptor dysfunction of unknown cause

VISUAL FIELD QUIZ

1. Test yourself in the interpretation of the following hypothetical cases (Exercises 1 to 33).

2. Unless stated otherwise, assume that the visual fields have been evaluated with a perimeter using the same stimulus and testing conditions for each eye.

3. Describe and categorize the visual field defects and suggest the probable localization and possible causes of the lesion(s).

4. Develop a systematic approach that includes a review of the "Ten Key Points to Remember."

5. Remember the significance of altered visual acuities (see Chapter 1, V, B, 6).

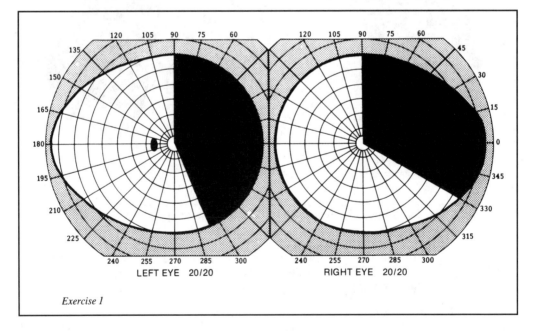

LEFT EYE   20/20   RIGHT EYE   20/20

Exercise 1

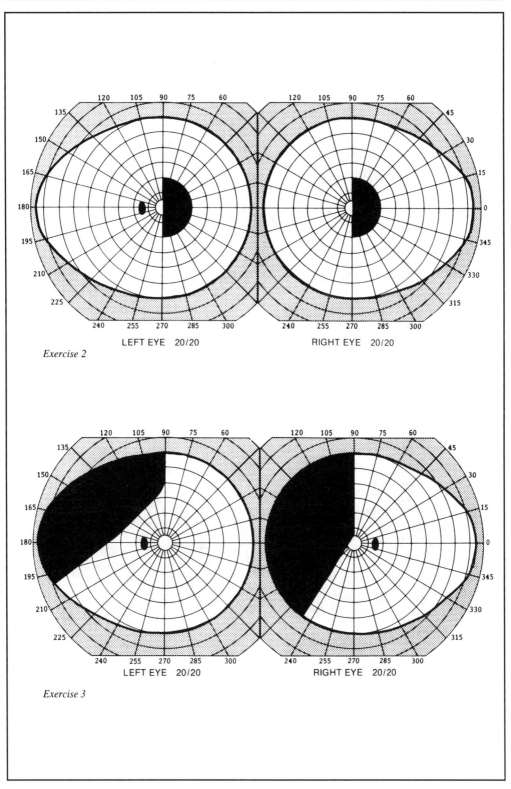

Exercise 2

LEFT EYE 20/20   RIGHT EYE 20/20

Exercise 3

LEFT EYE 20/20   RIGHT EYE 20/20

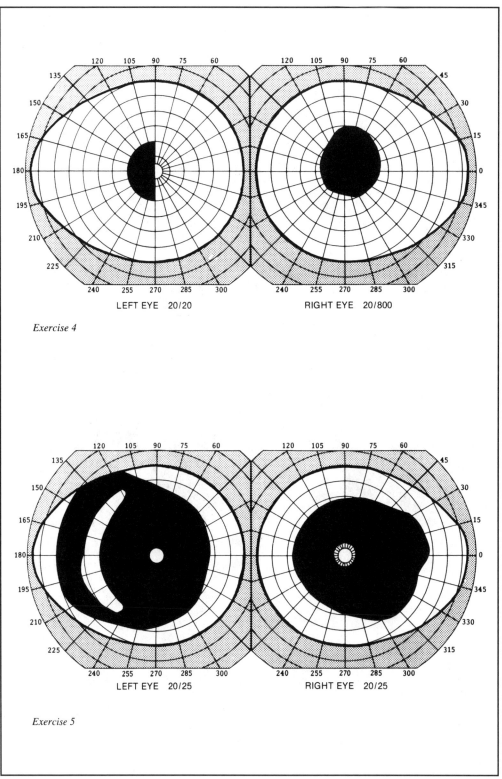

LEFT EYE   20/20   RIGHT EYE   20/800

Exercise 4

LEFT EYE   20/25   RIGHT EYE   20/25

Exercise 5

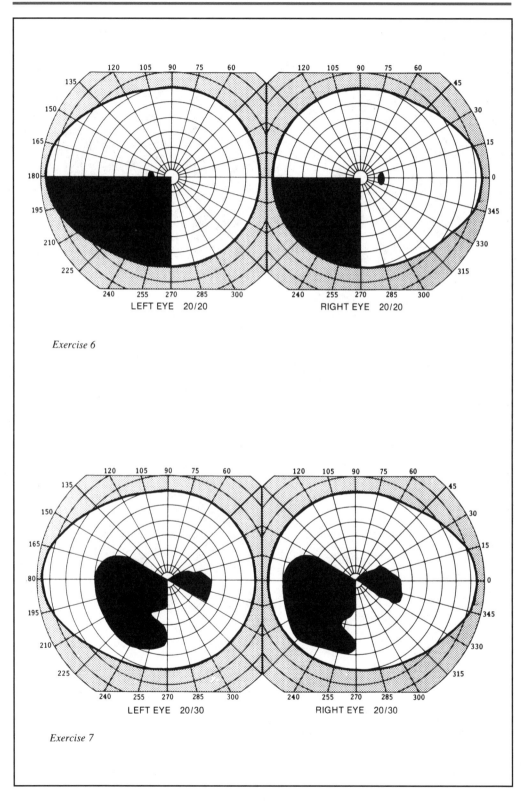

Exercise 6

Exercise 7

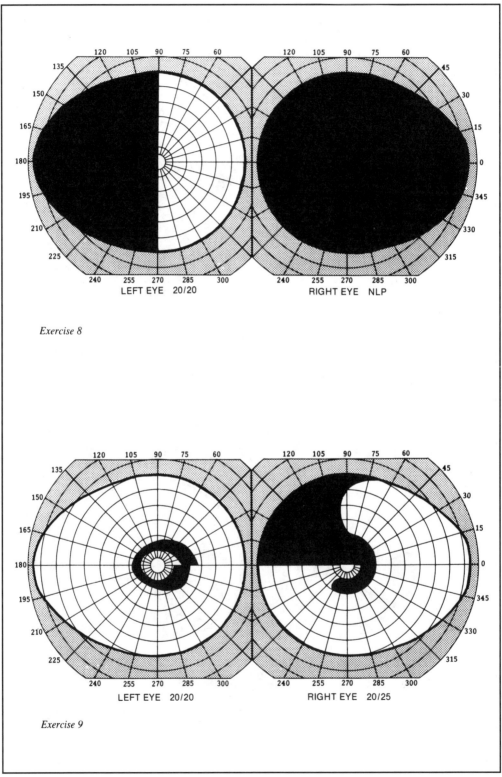

LEFT EYE 20/20

RIGHT EYE NLP

Exercise 8

LEFT EYE 20/20

RIGHT EYE 20/25

Exercise 9

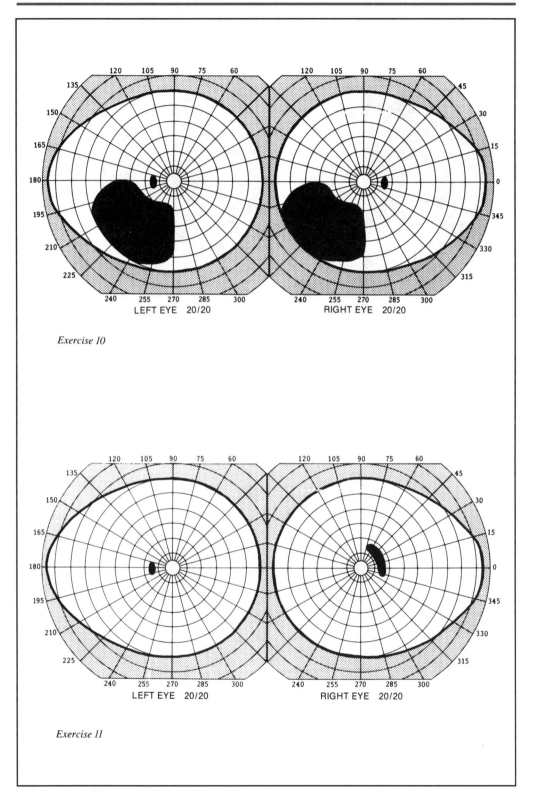

LEFT EYE 20/20

RIGHT EYE 20/20

Exercise 10

LEFT EYE 20/20

RIGHT EYE 20/20

Exercise 11

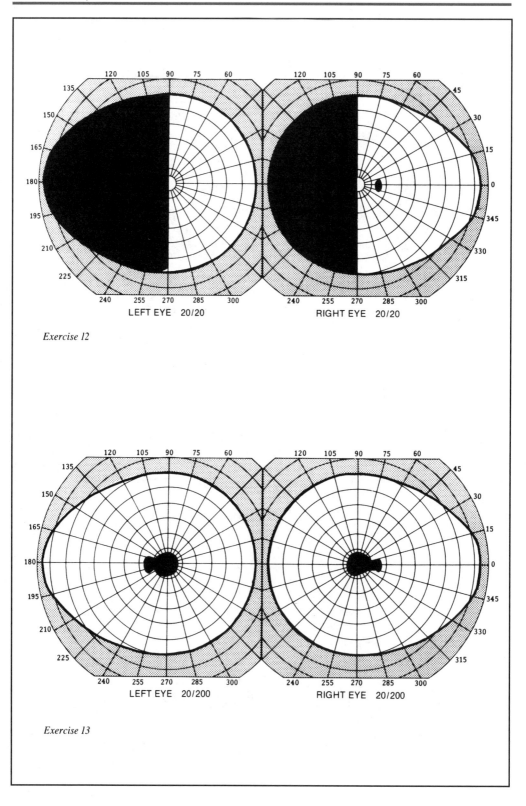

LEFT EYE   20/20

RIGHT EYE   20/20

Exercise 12

LEFT EYE   20/200

RIGHT EYE   20/200

Exercise 13

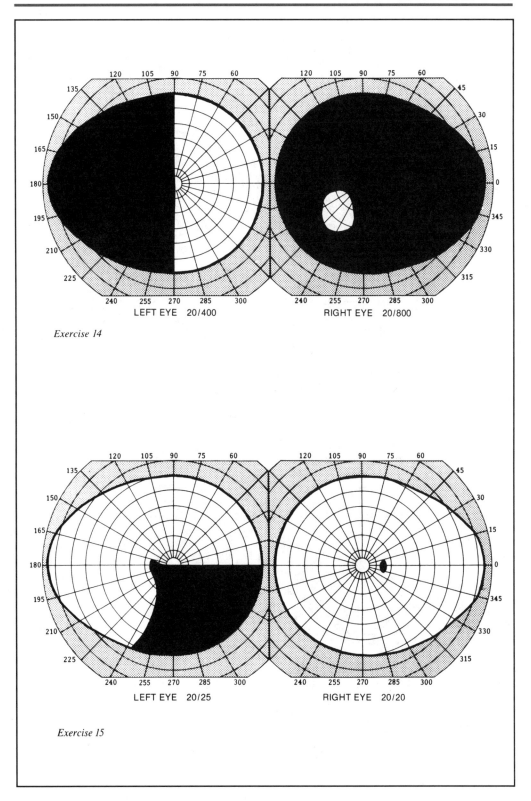

LEFT EYE 20/400

RIGHT EYE 20/800

Exercise 14

LEFT EYE 20/25

RIGHT EYE 20/20

Exercise 15

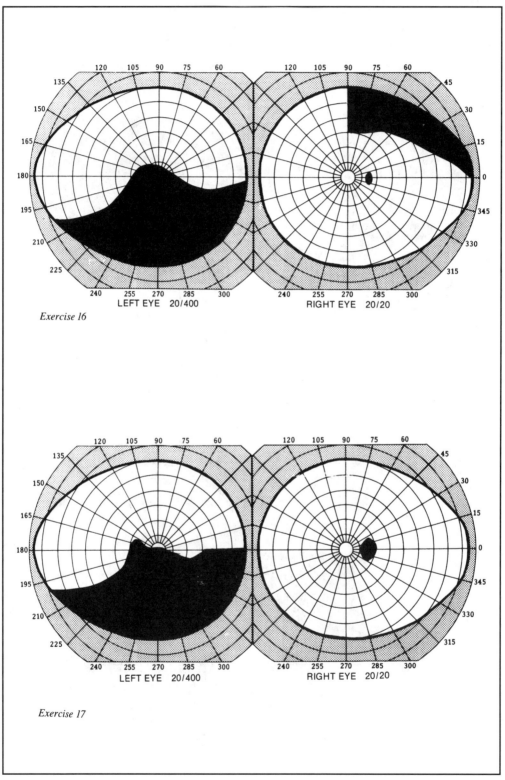

Exercise 16

Exercise 17

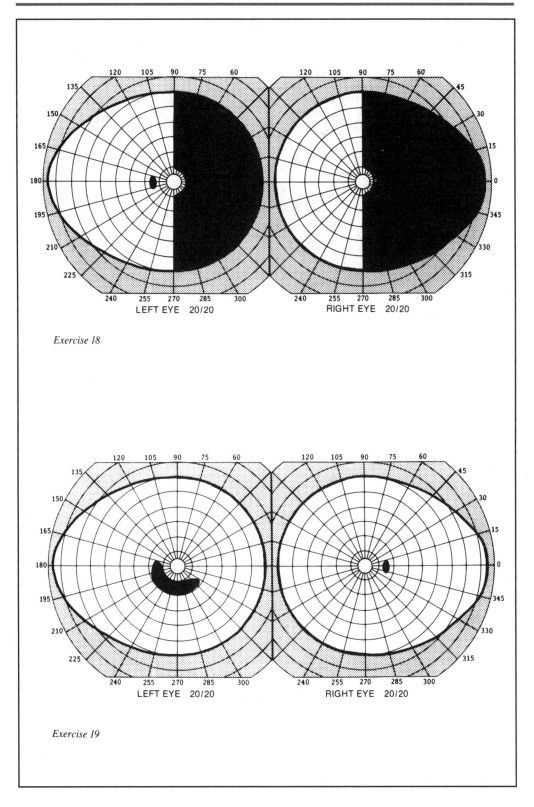

Exercise 18

LEFT EYE   20/20

RIGHT EYE   20/20

Exercise 19

LEFT EYE   20/20

RIGHT EYE   20/20

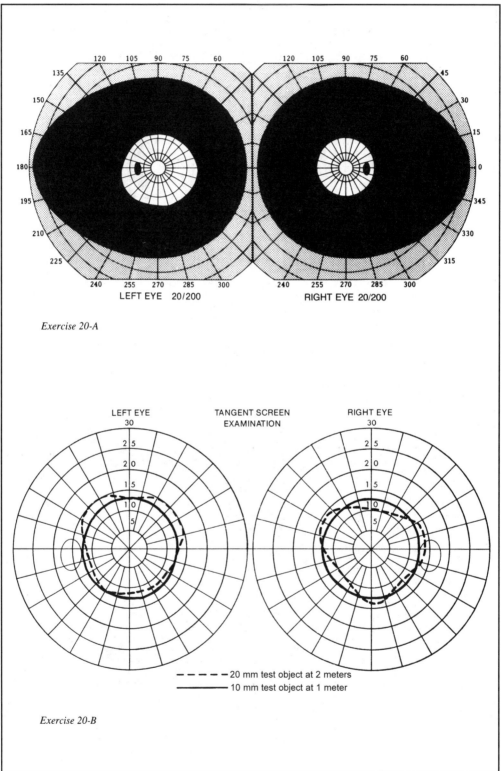

Exercise 20-A

LEFT EYE 20/200

RIGHT EYE 20/200

LEFT EYE
TANGENT SCREEN
EXAMINATION
RIGHT EYE

- - - - - 20 mm test object at 2 meters
———— 10 mm test object at 1 meter

Exercise 20-B

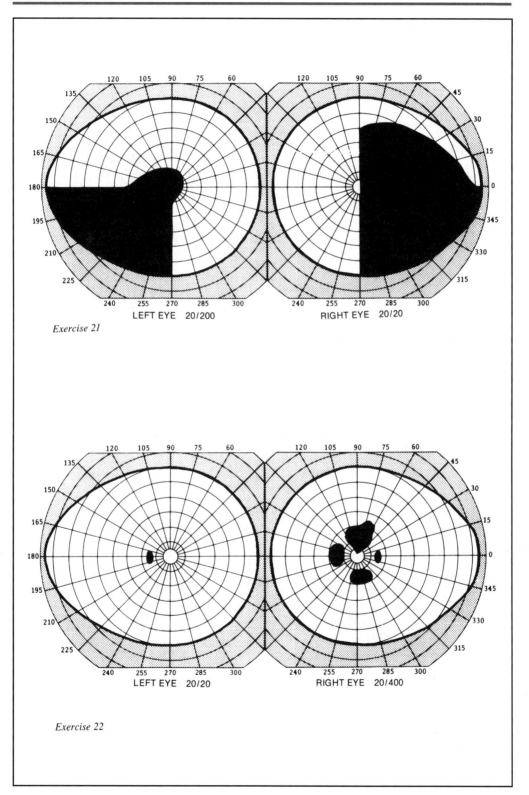

Exercise 21

LEFT EYE 20/200

RIGHT EYE 20/20

Exercise 22

LEFT EYE 20/20

RIGHT EYE 20/400

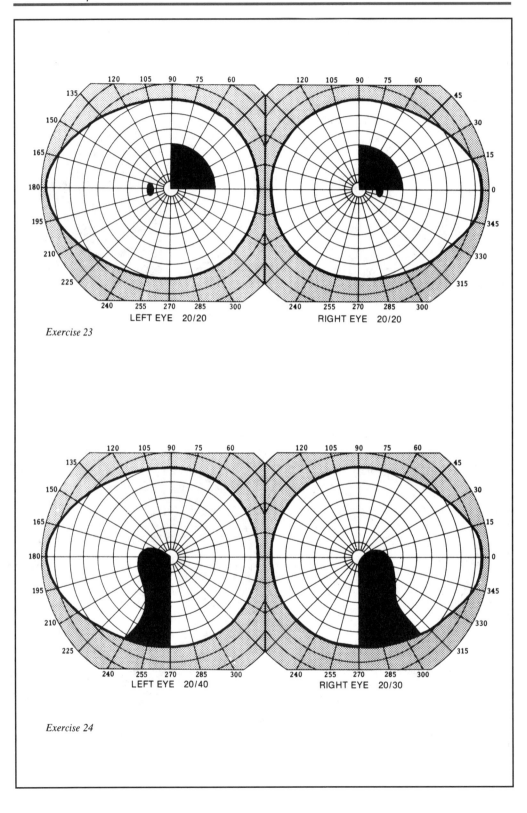

LEFT EYE   20/20   RIGHT EYE   20/20

Exercise 23

LEFT EYE   20/40   RIGHT EYE   20/30

Exercise 24

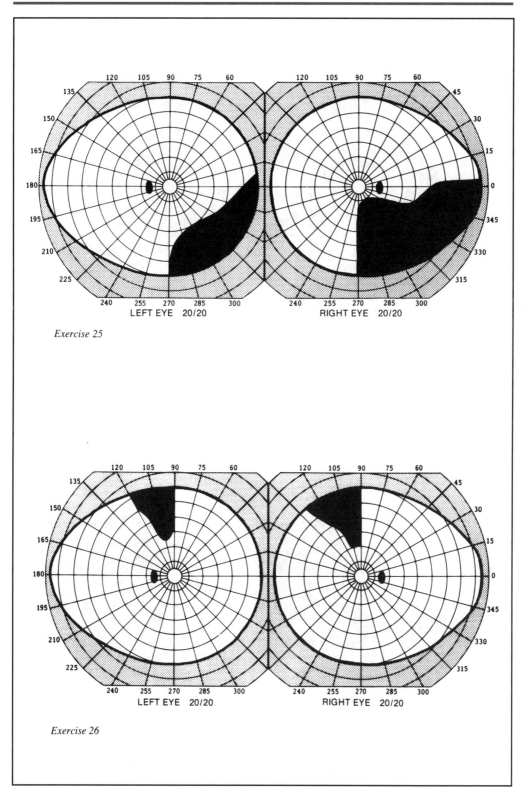

Exercise 25

LEFT EYE 20/20   RIGHT EYE 20/20

Exercise 26

LEFT EYE 20/20   RIGHT EYE 20/20

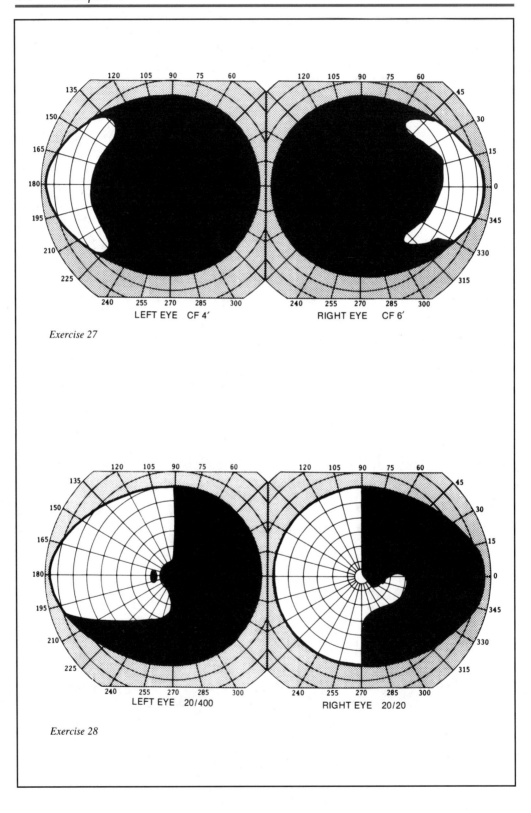

LEFT EYE   CF 4′   RIGHT EYE   CF 6′

Exercise 27

LEFT EYE   20/400   RIGHT EYE   20/20

Exercise 28

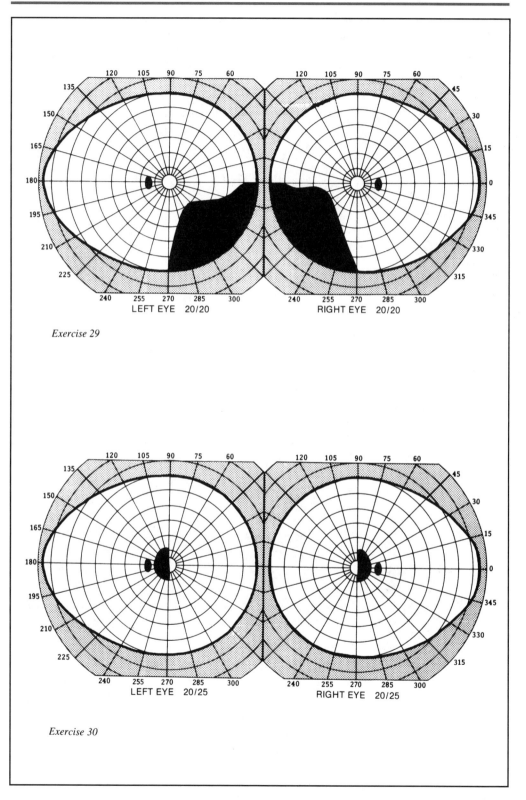

Exercise 29

Exercise 30

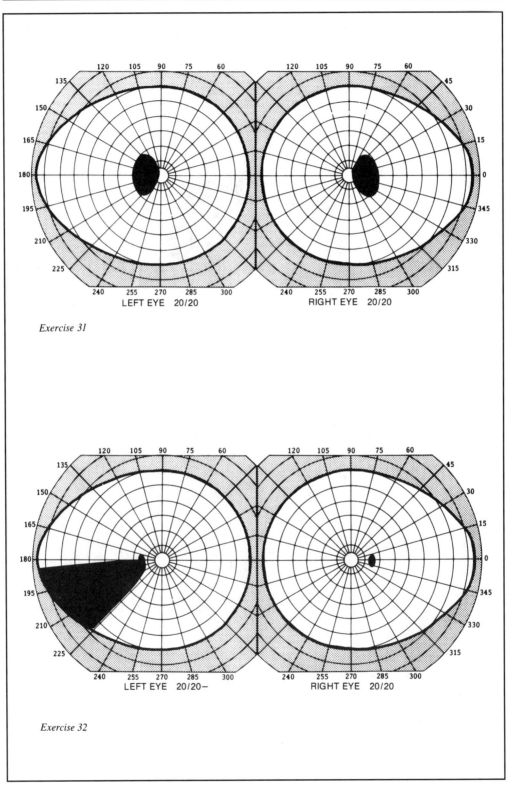

Exercise 31

Exercise 32

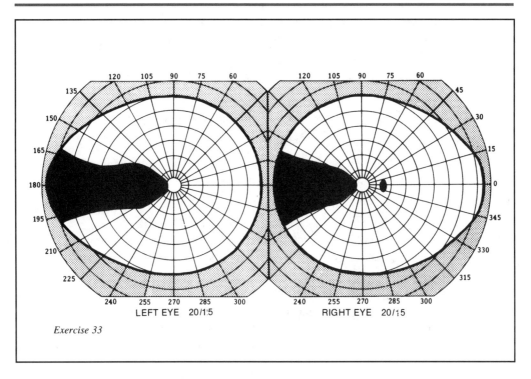

LEFT EYE   20/1'5   RIGHT EYE   20/15

Exercise 33

PLAUSIBLE INTERPRETATIONS
OF THE MYSTERY VISUAL FIELD DEFECTS

E1. R homonymous hemianopia, incongruous, denser above but extending to fixation and into the inferior quadrants. L temporal lobe lesion extending to the L parietal lobe.

E2. R homonymous hemianopia, central (macular), congruous. L occipital tip.

E3. L homonymous hemianopia, denser above, markedly incongruous. Marked incongruity suggests possibility of R optic tract lesion, but greater density above suggests possibility of R temporal lobe lesion, which would also be 10 times more likely statistically.

E4. R central scotoma; L central (macular) temporal hemianopia. R optic nerve lesion at the junction of the nerve and chiasm.

E5. Bilateral ring scotomas with preservation of central 10 to 20 degrees with vision of 20/25 OU. Retinitis pigmentosa vs advanced glaucoma.

E6. L homonymous inferior quadrantanopia, congruous. R parietal vs occipital lesion. The congruity gives the edge to the occipital localization.

E7. Bilateral incomplete homonymous hemianopias, congruous. Bilateral occipital lesions.

E8. Blind OD with temporal hemianopia OS. R optic nerve lesion extending into the chiasm.

E9. Superior and inferior arcuate defects OS, creating a "ring" scotoma. OD: inferior arcuate scotoma and larger, superior arcuate scotoma breaking through nasally to create a nasal step. Glaucoma.

E10. L homonymous inferior quadrantanopia, congruous, with sparing of temporal crescent OS, and bilateral macular sparing. R occipital lesion, upper bank of the calcarine fissure.

El1. R superior nerve fiber layer defect (Seidel scotoma). Glaucoma. Expect to see inferior elongation of the right cup.

E12. L homonymous hemianopia, complete (cannot make statement about congruity). R optic tract, parietal, or occipital lesion. OKN asymmetry would identify the parietal cases.

E13. Bilateral centrocecal scotomas. Bilateral optic neuropathy.

E14. Inferior nasal island remaining OD. Temporal hemianopia with involvement of central field OS. Extensive chiasmatic lesion.

E15. Inferior NFB defect OS. OD normal. OS optic nerve lesion: glaucoma vs ischemic optic neuropathy.

E16. Inferior NFB (altitudinal) defect OS with involvement of central field. Superior temporal cut OD. Lesion at junction of L optic nerve and chiasm (junctional scotoma).

E17. Inferior NFB (altitudinal) defect OS with involvement of the central field. Enlarged blind spot OD. Intracranial left optic nerve lesion. Be suspicious that the lesion is intracranial because the right optic disc appears to be edematous, probably due to increased intracranial pressure caused by the left optic nerve tumor (meningioma). Expect to see the disc changes associated with the Foster Kennedy syndrome (optic atrophy OS and disc edema OD).

E18. R homonymous hemianopia, complete, with macular sparing. L occipital cortex.

E19. Inferior arcuate scotoma (NFB defect) OS. OD normal. Look for disc changes. Superior elongation of the cup (glaucoma). Lumpy disc (drusen).

E20. Tubular fields with discrepancy of size of remaining fields when comparing perimeter (20-A) and tangent screen (20-B) fields. "Tunnel" vision. Non-organic field defects.

E21. Bitemporal hemianopia with central scotoma OS. Chiasm.

E22. Multiple central and paracentral defects OD. OS normal. Retinal lesions (chorioretinitis).

E23. R homonymous superior quadrantanopia, congruous, central, involving macular field. L occipital tip, inferior calcarine cortex.

E24. Inferior bitemporal hemianopia. Chiasmatic lesion with some involvement of the macular fibers, causing slightly decreased acuities.

E25. R homonymous, inferior quadrantanopia, markedly incongruous. L parietal vs L optic tract.

E26. L homonymous superior quadrantanopia incongruous. "Pie in the sky" defects. R temporal lobe (Meyer's loop) lesion.

E27. Temporal islands remaining OU. Endstage glaucoma.

E28. R homonymous hemianopia, incongruous, with central scotoma OS. L optic tract lesion at junction of tract and chiasm, affecting some of the crossing macular fibers of the left eye, causing decreased acuity in that eye.

E29. Bilateral inferior nasal contraction. Optic nerve or retinal lesions (optic disc drusen, glaucoma, retinoschisis).

E30. Bitemporal hemianopia, central (macular). Chiasm.

E31. Enlarged blind spots OU, causing pseudobitemporal (central) hemianopia: papilledema.

E32. Inferior-temporal wedge-shaped field defect OS. OD normal. A NFB defect affecting the superior-nasal bundle of nerve fibers (see Figures 1-7 and 1-9). An uncommon but well-documented glaucomatous field defect. May also represent the residual of optic neuritis.

E33. Congruous horizontal wedge-shaped left homonymous, horizontal sectoranopia. A rare field defect due to a lesion of right LGN.

BIBLIOGRAPHY

Books

Anderson DR. *Perimetry: With and Without Automation*. 2nd ed. St Louis, Mo: CV Mosby; 1987.

Bundez PL. *Atlas of Visual Fields*. Philadelphia, Pa: Lippincott-Raven; 1997.

Traquair HM. *Clinical Perimetry*. 7th ed. London: Henry Kimpton; 1957.

Walsh TJ, ed. Visual fields: examination and interpretation. *Ophthalmology Monographs*. Vol 3. San Francisco, Calif: American Academy of Ophthalmology; 1996.

Chapters

Glaser JS. *Neuro-Ophthalmology*. 3rd ed. Philadelphia, Pa: Lippincott Williams & Wilkins; 1999:5-7.

Sadun AA, Agarwal MR. Topical diagnosis of acquired optic nerve disorders. In: Miller NR, Newman NJ, eds. *Walsh and Hoyt's Clinical Neuro-Ophthalmology*. 6th ed. Vol 1. Philadelphia, Pa: Lippincott Williams & Wilkins; 2005:197-236.

Articles

Barton JJS, Hefter R, Chang B, et al. The field defects of anterior temporal lobectomy: a quantitative reassessment of Meyer's loop. *Brain*. 2005;128:2123-2133.

Donahue SP, Kardon RH, Thompson HS. Hourglass-shaped visual fields as a sign of bilateral lateral geniculate myelinolysis. *Am J Ophthalmol*. 1995;119:378-379.

Frisén L. Quadruple sectoranopia and sectorial optic atrophy: a syndrome of the distal anterior choroidal artery. *J Neurol Neurosurg Psychiatry*. 1979;42:590-594.

Frisén L, Holmegeard L, Rosencrantz M. Sectorial optic atrophy and homonymous, horizontal sectoranopia: a lateral choroidal artery syndrome? *J Neurol Neurosurg Psychiatry*. 1978;41:374-380.

Hershenfeld SA, Sharpe JA. Monocular temporal hemianopia. *Br J Ophthalmol*. 1993;77:424-427.

Horton JC. Wilbrand's knee of the primate chiasm is an artifact of monocular enucleation. *Trans Am Ophthalmol Soc*. 1997;95:579-609.

Horton JC, Hoyt WF. The representation of the visual field in human striate cortex. A revision of the classic Holmes map. *Arch Ophthalmol*. 1991;109:816-824.

Hoyt WF, Luis O. The primate chiasm: details of visual fiber organization studied by silver impregnation techniques. *Arch Ophthalmol*. 1962;68:94-106.

Hoyt WF, Tudor RC. The course of parapapillary temporal retinal axons through the anterior optic nerve. A Nanta degeneration study in the primate. *Arch Ophthalmol*. 1963;69:503-507.

Karanjia N, Jacobson DM. Compression of the prechiasmatic optic nerve produces a junctional scotoma. *Am J Ophthalmol*. 1999;128:256-258.

Quillen DA, Davis JA, Gottlieb JL. The white dot syndromes. *Am J Ophthalmol.* 2004;137:538-550.

Savino PJ, Paris M, Schatz NJ, et al. Optic tract syndrome. *Arch Ophthalmol.* 1978;96:656-663.

Smith JL, Cogan DG. Optokinetic nystagmus: a test for parietal lobe lesions. *Am J Ophthalmol.* 1959;48:187-193.

Smith TJ, Baker RS. Perimetric findings in functional disorders using automated techniques. *Ophthalmology.* 1987;94:1562-1566.

Watzke RC, Shults WT. Clinical features and natural history of the acute idiopathic enlarged blind spot syndrome. *Ophthalmology.* 2002;109:1326-1335.

Zhang X, Kedar S, Lynn MJ, et al. Homonymous hemianopias: clinical-anatomic correlations in 904 cases. *Neurology.* 2006;66:906-910.

Chapter 2

Supranuclear and Internuclear Gaze Pathways

Mark F. Walker, MD, and Lanning B. Kline, MD

I. **Six types of eye movements, five conjugate and one disconjugate, and the fixation system control the position of the fovea (Table 2-1)**

   A. Saccades and quick phases direct the fovea to a new location in the visual scene

   B. Pursuit, optokinetic slow phases, and vestibular slow phases stabilize images on the fovea

   C. Vergence moves the eyes in opposite directions to realign the two foveas

II. **Functional classification of eye movements**

   A. Saccades

      1. Purpose: to shift gaze (the fovea) to a new location in the visual scene
      2. Stimuli
         a. Sudden appearance of a new stimulus (visual, auditory, somatosensory): reflexive saccade (look toward a possible threat)
         b. Voluntary change in gaze direction to another point in an already visible scene: voluntary saccade (eg, visual scanning)
      3. Saccades are very fast, and the speed of the saccade depends on its size (bigger saccades are faster)
      4. Visual "suppression" during saccades: even though the visual world is sweeping rapidly across the retina, there is no sense of a blurred image

   B. Quick phases

      1. Purpose: to reset the position of the eyes during nystagmus, so that they do not reach an extreme orbital position
      2. Quick phases are very similar to saccades, for which they are the phylogenetic forerunner

   C. Pursuit

      1. Purpose: to allow the fovea to maintain fixation of a moving target
      2. Stimuli
         a. Motion of the image of a target across the foveal and parafoveal retina (retinal slip)

Table 2-1

EYE MOVEMENT

Type	Function
Conjugate Eye Movements	
Saccades	Redirect the fovea
Quick phases of nystagmus	Reset eye position toward the oncoming visual scene
Pursuit	Tracks a moving object
Vestibular slow phases	Keep image on the fovea when the head is moving
Optokinetic slow phases	Tracks full-field visual motion
Disconjugate Eye Movements	
Vergence	Aligns both foveas on the same object in the visual scene

b.   Nonvisual stimuli, such as proprioception, can also evoke pursuit (eg, following one's own fingers in darkness)

3.   When a target starts moving, the eyes first accelerate (over about 100 ms) to the target speed, then track it by matching eye speed to target speed

4.   Pursuit gain is defined as the ratio of eye speed to target speed

5.   If the eyes cannot keep up with the target (either because the target is moving too fast or because pursuit is deficient), then catch-up saccades bring the foveas back on target, leading to jerky-appearing saccadic pursuit

D.   Optokinetic responses

1.   Purpose: to stabilize the visual image on the retina, when the whole visual scene is moving

2.   Stimulus: motion of the entire visual scene across the retina due to prolonged self-motion (eg, looking out of the window while riding on a train)

3.   The optokinetic system supplements vestibular responses during prolonged motion

E.   Vestibulo-ocular reflex (VOR)

1.   Purpose: the VOR generates an eye movement in the direction opposite to that of the head motion, in order to keep the stationary visual image stable on the retina, maintaining clear vision when the head moves

2.   Stimuli: the vestibular system is activated by two types of head motion: rotations and translations (linear motion)

3.   Head motion is sensed by the vestibular labyrinth of the inner ear

a.   The three semicircular canals (horizontal or lateral, anterior or superior, posterior) sense head rotations

b.   The two otolith organs (utricle and saccule) sense head translations

4.   The compensatory eye movement of the VOR is called a "slow phase," although it can be fast (>200 degrees/sec) if the head is rotating quickly

5.   Failure of the VOR leads to oscillopsia (the illusion that the world is moving) during head motion

F. Vergence

    1. Purpose: vergence eye movements realign the foveas on a new object at a different depth (viewing distance)

    2. Stimuli:

        a. Different positions of the image of an object on the retinas of the two eyes (retinal disparity). This leads to fusional vergence

        b. Loss of focus of images on the retina (retinal blur). This leads to accommodative vergence

    3. Vergence movements are disconjugate: they rotate the eyes in opposite directions

    4. Vergence eye movements can be horizontal (convergence, divergence), vertical, or torsional (excyclovergence, incyclovergence)

G. Fixation

    1. Purpose: the fixation system is an additional system that keeps the eyes still in the orbits to maintain gaze when neither the head nor the object is moving

III. Neural pathways for eye movements (Figure 2-1)

A. Saccade pathways

    1. Mediated by parallel pathways (Figure 2-2)

        a. Frontal cortex—frontal eye field (FEF), supplementary eye field, dorsolateral prefrontal cortex (to the superior colliculus [SC] and directly to the brainstem saccade generators [BSGs])

        b. Posterior parietal cortex (PPC) to the SC

    2. The frontocollicular pathway generates voluntary saccades, and the parietocollicular pathway generates reflexive saccades to novel targets

    3. Horizontal saccades

        a. Originate in the FEF and PPC, contralateral to the saccade direction (eg, the right FEF and PPC generate leftward saccades)

        b. Cortical saccade neurons project to the SC on the same side. The FEF also projects to the BSG directly and through the basal ganglia. This allows for saccades to be preserved if the SC is lesioned

        c. Natural or electrical stimulation of the SC elicits a contraversive saccade. The SC has a topographic map; each position corresponds to a saccade of a particular size and direction

        d. The SC projects to the BSG on the opposite side

        e. The BSG converts the spatial code of the SC signal (specifying the saccade vector) to a rate code (the innervation signal for the ocular motor neurons)

        f. The saccade signal consists of two elements (Figure 2-3)

            i. A high-frequency burst (the pulse) immediately preceding the saccade overcomes orbital viscosity to move the eye quickly to its new position. The pulse is generated by the burst neurons. Without a pulse, the eyes move very slowly

            ii. A new tonic signal (the step) provides the appropriate innervation to hold the eyes at the new position against elastic restoring forces. The step is generated by integrating the pulse (the neural integrator). Without a step, the eye drifts back to the center of the orbit

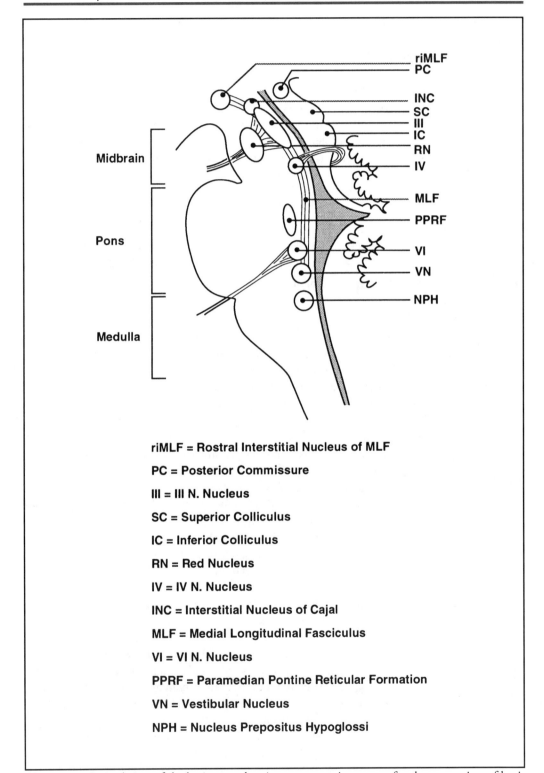

riMLF = Rostral Interstitial Nucleus of MLF

PC = Posterior Commissure

III = III N. Nucleus

SC = Superior Colliculus

IC = Inferior Colliculus

RN = Red Nucleus

IV = IV N. Nucleus

INC = Interstitial Nucleus of Cajal

MLF = Medial Longitudinal Fasciculus

VI = VI N. Nucleus

PPRF = Paramedian Pontine Reticular Formation

VN = Vestibular Nucleus

NPH = Nucleus Prepositus Hypoglossi

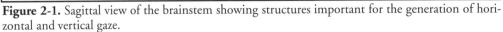

Figure 2-1. Sagittal view of the brainstem showing structures important for the generation of horizontal and vertical gaze.

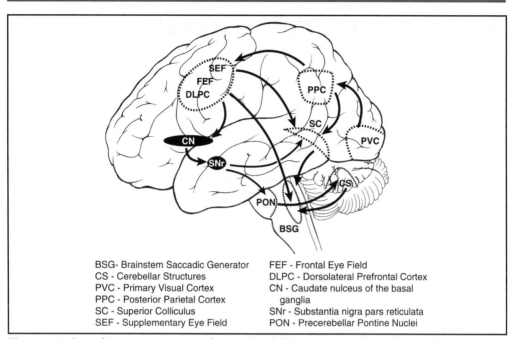

Figure 2-2. Saccadic eye movement pathways. Cerebellar structures (CS) of particular importance include the vermis and fastigial nucleus.

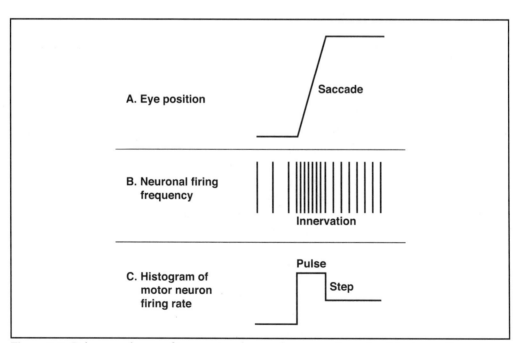

Figure 2-3. Pulse-step change of innervation that produces saccades and quick phases of nystagmus. Ocular motor neurons generate a high frequency discharge (pulse) that moves the eye at high velocity, followed by a tonic discharge (step) that maintains the desired eye position.

Table 2-2		

BRAINSTEM SACCADE GENERATORS

	Horizontal Saccades	**Vertical Saccades**
Burst neurons	Paramedian pontine reticular formation (PPRF)	Rostral interstitial nucleus of the medial longitudinal fasciculus (riMLF)
Integrator	Nucleus prepositus hypoglossi (NPH) and medial vestibular nucleus (MVN)	Interstitial nucleus of Cajal (INC)

g. There are separate saccade generators for horizontal and vertical saccades (Table 2-2)

h. The cerebellar vermis, through the fastigial nucleus, adjusts innervation to maintain saccade accuracy and adapt to changes (eg, extraocular muscle weakness)

4. Vertical saccades

a. Cortical pathways descend to the rostral interstitial nucleus of the medial longitudinal fasciculus (riMLF) in the midbrain just rostral to the oculomotor (CN III) nucleus at the junction of the midbrain and thalamus

b. Bilateral FEF or SC stimulation is required to elicit purely vertical saccades

c. There are different pathways for upward and downward saccades: upward burst neurons in the riMLF project bilaterally, whereas downward burst neurons project only ipsilaterally (Figure 2-4)

B. Pursuit pathways

1. Although classically viewed as distinct, new data are suggesting that there is substantial overlap between the brain areas controlling pursuit and saccades

2. Several cortical areas are involved in pursuit (Figure 2-5)

a. Medial temporal (MT) and medial superior temporal (MST) cortex: these areas at the parieto-temporal-occipital junction process visual motion signals that drive pursuit

b. FEF: lesions dramatically reduce pursuit gain

c. Posterior parietal cortex (PPC)

d. The cerebral cortex primarily controls ipsiversive pursuit (opposite to saccades). Hemispheric lesions generally impair pursuit toward the side of the lesion

e. Pure occipital lesions cause homonymous hemianopia, but patients can generally pursue in either direction, as long as the target is in the intact visual hemifield

f. Parietal lesions may also cause akinetopsia (impaired motion perception)

g. Because several cerebellar structures are important for pursuit (see Figure 2-5), diffuse cerebellar disease severely impairs pursuit

    C.   Optokinetic slow-phases

        1.   In afoveates, optokinetic responses are elicited via the accessory optic system through retinal projections to the nucleus of the optic tract in the pretectum

        2.   In humans, responses to full-field visual motion likely involve both cortical and subcortical mechanisms

    D.   Vergence

        1.   Visual signals from occipital cortex project to vergence premotor neurons in the midbrain reticular formation (MRF)

        2.   Three types of premotor neurons in the MRF:

            a.   Vergence tonic cells: discharge in relation to vergence angle

            b.   Vergence burst cells: discharge in relation to vergence velocity

            c.   Vergence burst-tonic cells: combine position and velocity signals

        3.   Premotor neurons project to the oculomotor (CN III) nuclear complex to elicit the near triad: convergence, accommodation, miosis

IV.   Binocular coordination

    A.   Most eye movements (except for vergence) are conjugate—the eyes move together in the same direction by roughly the same amount. To accomplish this, the brain must coordinate the movements of the two eyes

    B.   Horizontal eye movements are coordinated through the projection of abducens interneurons via the medial longitudinal fasciculus (MLF) to contralateral medial rectus (MR) motoneurons (Figure 2-6)

        1.   Premotor commands for horizontal saccades (in the paramedian pontine reticular formation [PPRF]) and horizontal pursuit (from the vestibular nuclei) are sent to the adjacent abducens nucleus, to both abducens motoneurons and abducens interneurons

        2.   Abducens motoneurons innervate the ipsilateral lateral rectus, leading to abduction

        3.   Abducens interneurons send their axons across the midline to the contralateral MLF, where they ascend to the oculomotor nucleus (CN III), synapsing on MR motoneurons

        4.   Thus, there is a coordinated abduction of one eye and adduction of the other eye

    C.   Vertical eye movements are coordinated in the midbrain

        1.   Burst neurons (riMLF) and tonic neurons (interstitial nucleus of Cajal [INC]) project directly to motoneurons of yoked muscles (eg, right SR and left IO). This differs from the horizontal system, where the eyes are yoked by abducens interneurons

        2.   The SR and SO muscles have crossed innervation (eg, the left trochlear nucleus innervates the right SO muscle). This facilitates binocular coordination, because cell bodies innervating yoked muscles (eg, right SO and left IR muscles) are on the same side of the brainstem (left)

V.   VOR

    A.   The VOR generates an eye movement in the opposite direction as the head movement, of the appropriate speed to keep the visual image of the external world still on the retina as the head moves

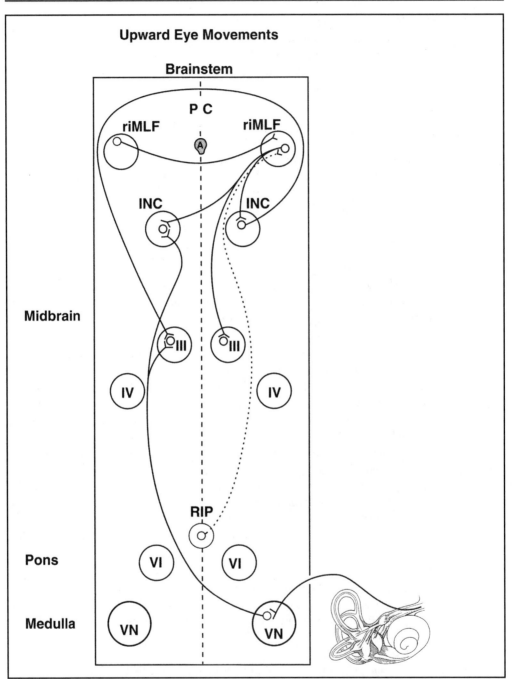

Figure 2-4 (left). Brainstem pathways for vertical gaze, upward (left) and downward (right, opposite page). Vestibular inputs from the vertical semicircular canals synapse in the vestibular nucleus and ascend in the contralateral MLF and brachium conjunctivum (not shown) to contact neurons in IV, III, INC, and riMLF. The riMLF contains saccadic burst neurons and receives an inhibitory input from omnipause neurons of the nucleus raphe interpositus (RIP). Excitatory burst neurons in the riMLF project to III, IV, and send an axon collateral to INC. The INC provides a gaze-holding signal and projects to vertical motoneurons via the posterior commissure (PC). A=aqueduct of Sylvius. (Modified from Leigh RJ, Zee DS. *The Neurology of Eye Movements.* 3rd ed. New York, NY: Oxford University Press; 1999:225.)

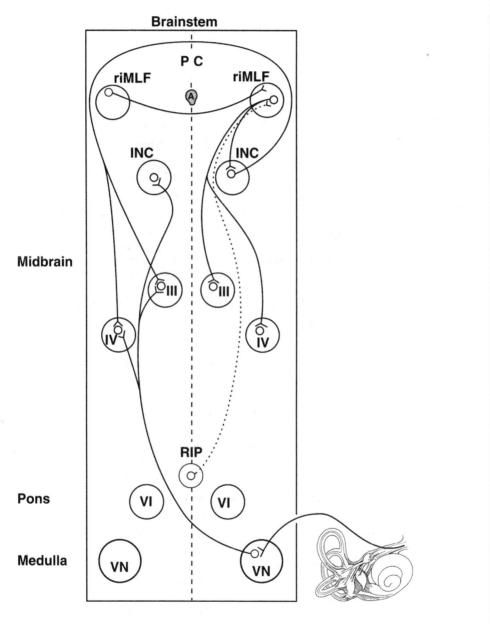

Figure 2-4 (right).

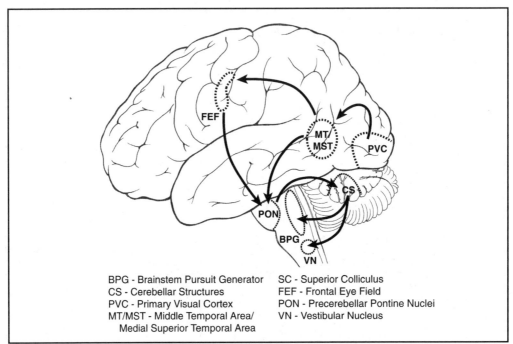

BPG - Brainstem Pursuit Generator   SC - Superior Colliculus
CS - Cerebellar Structures   FEF - Frontal Eye Field
PVC - Primary Visual Cortex   PON - Precerebellar Pontine Nuclei
MT/MST - Middle Temporal Area/   VN - Vestibular Nucleus
    Medial Superior Temporal Area

Figure 2-5. Pursuit eye movement pathways. Cerebellar structures (CS) of particular importance include vermis, flocculus, and paraflocculus.

B.   Head motion is sensed by the vestibular labyrinth (Figure 2-7)

1.   The three semicircular canals (horizontal or lateral, anterior or superior, posterior) sense head rotations

2.   The two otolith organs (utricle, saccule) sense head orientation relative to gravity and linear motion of the head

3.   "Labyrinth-within-a-labyrinth": The membranous labyrinth (filled with potassium-rich endolymph) sits within the bony labyrinth (filled with CSF-like perilymph) in the petrous portion of the temporal bone

C.   Each semicircular canal has a particular orientation that determines the direction of the rotations that stimulate it. The three canals are roughly orthogonal to each other (Figure 2-8)

1.   The horizontal canals (HC) are located in a plane that is tilted about 30 degrees up from the earth-horizontal plane. Each HC is excited by a rotation toward it and inhibited by a rotation away from it (eg, rightward rotation excites the right HC and inhibits the left HC)

2.   The anterior (AC) and posterior (PC) canals are each oriented about midway between the sagittal and coronal planes

3.   The canals are arranged in three pairs (RHC-LHC, RAC-LPC, LAC-RPC), each of which is roughly in a common plane. These canals operate in a "push-pull" fashion: a given rotation excites one canal in the pair and inhibits the other

4.   Each canal pair is associated with a pair of extraocular muscles that lies roughly in the same plane (Figures 2-9a through 2-9c, Table 2-3)

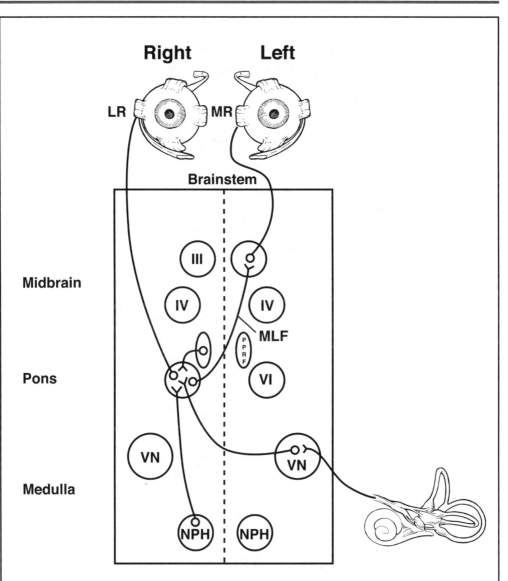

Figure 2-6. Brainstem pathways for horizontal gaze. Axons from cell bodies in the PPRF travel to ipsilateral VI where they synapse with abducens motoneurons, axons of which travel to ipsilateral lateral rectus (LR). Abducens internuclear neurons have axons that cross the midline and travel in the MLF to contact medial rectus (MR) motoneurons in contralateral III. Eye position information (neural integrator) reaches VI from neurons within the nucleus prepositus hypoglossi (NPH) and vestibular nuclei (VN). (Modified from Leigh RJ, Zee DS. *The Neurology of Eye Movements.* 3rd ed. New York, NY: Oxford University Press; 1999:216.)

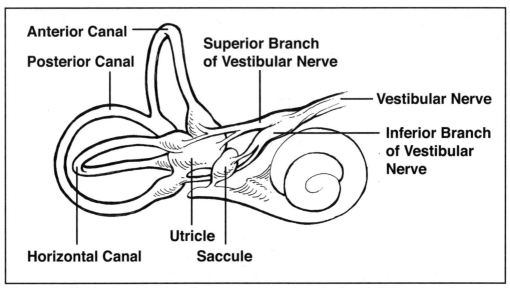

Figure 2-7. Membranous labyrinth of inner ear. Superior branch of vestibular nerve innervates anterior canal, horizontal canal, and utricle. Inferior branch innervates posterior canal and saccule.

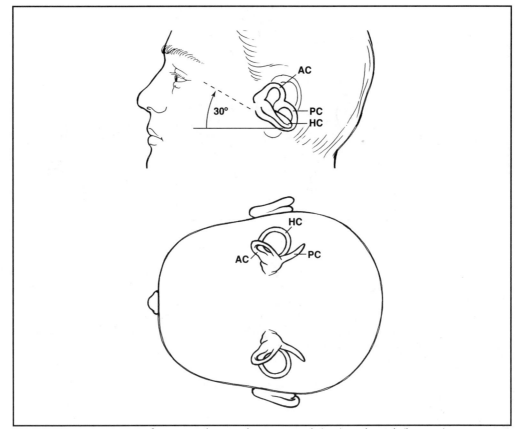

Figure 2-8. Orientation of semicircular canals on sagittal (top) and axial (bottom) projections. AC=anterior canal, HC=horizontal canal, PC=posterior canal.

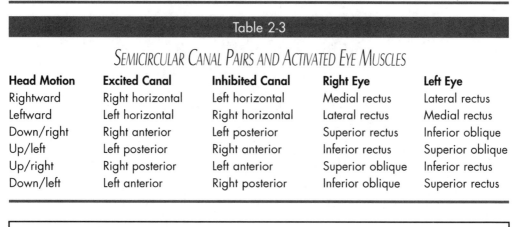

Head Motion	Excited Canal	Inhibited Canal	Right Eye	Left Eye
Rightward	Right horizontal	Left horizontal	Medial rectus	Lateral rectus
Leftward	Left horizontal	Right horizontal	Lateral rectus	Medial rectus
Down/right	Right anterior	Left posterior	Superior rectus	Inferior oblique
Up/left	Left posterior	Right anterior	Inferior rectus	Superior oblique
Up/right	Right posterior	Left anterior	Superior oblique	Inferior rectus
Down/left	Left anterior	Right posterior	Inferior oblique	Superior rectus

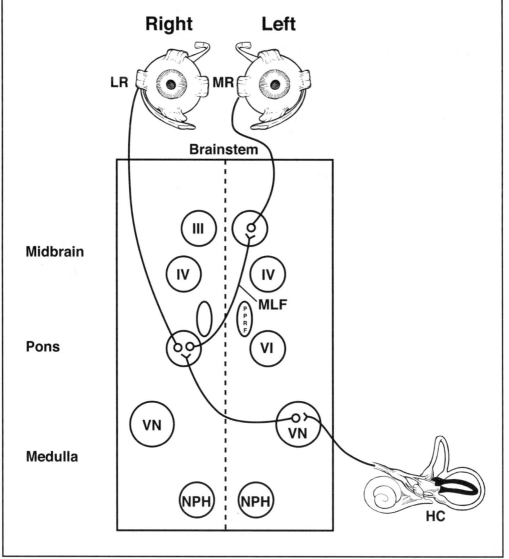

Figure 2-9a. Excitatory connections between horizontal semicircular canal and yoked extraocular muscles.

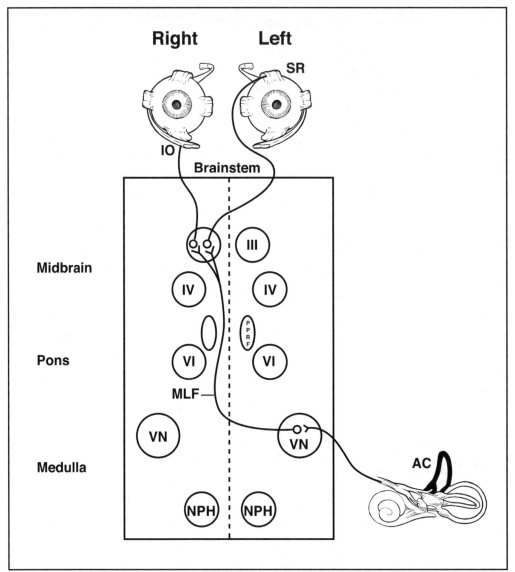

Figure 2-9b. Excitatory connections between anterior semicircular canal and yoked extraocular muscles.

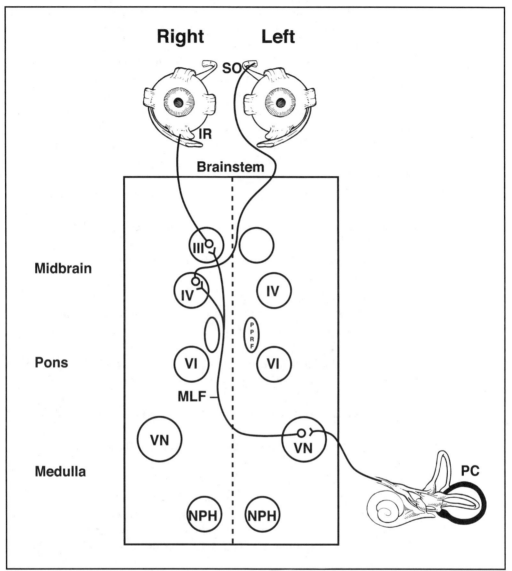

Figure 2-9c. Excitatory connections between posterior semicircular canal and yoked extraocular muscles.

5. The basic pathway of the VOR is a "three-neuron arc": primary vestibular afferent, secondary vestibular neuron, extraocular motoneuron (see Figures 2-9a through 2-9c)

6. When the head rotates, inertia of the endolymph causes it to lag behind, resulting in a relative motion of endolymph within the membranous canal (eg, rightward rotation leads to leftward endolymph motion)

7. At one end of each canal is a membrane called the cupula. Endolymph motion bows the cupula, causing deflection of hair cell stereocilia

8. A change in hair cell potential is transmitted to the vestibular afferent, which changes its firing rate up or down, depending on whether the rotation is in the excitatory or inhibitory direction

9. The vestibular afferent projects to secondary vestibular neurons in the vestibular nuclei

10. Secondary neurons project to the ocular motor nuclei (eg, abducens for the horizontal VOR)

11. Binocular gaze pathways ensure that movements of the two eyes are coordinated

D. Vestibular imbalance produces nystagmus

1. Each vestibular nerve has a resting discharge rate (~100 spikes/sec)

2. When the head is not moving, both vestibular nerves are discharging at the same rate (balanced)

3. When the head rotates, the discharge rate increases on one side and decreases on the other (eg, rightward rotation leads to an increased firing rate of the right vestibular nerve and a decreased rate of the left vestibular nerve)

4. The imbalance in vestibular nerve inputs tells the brain that the head is moving

5. The VOR generates a compensatory eye movement (the slow phase)

6. Quick phases in the opposite direction reset the position of the eyes and keep them from reaching extreme positions in the orbit

7. The combination of slow and quick phases is nystagmus

8. Nystagmus is often described by the direction of its quick phases, even though the slow phases are what really indicate what is happening in the vestibular system (eg, rightward rotation elicits leftward slow phases and a right-beating nystagmus)

E. Clinical testing of vestibular function

1. Head rotation

    a. The "doll's eye" maneuver (Figure 2-10): the examiner moves the head back and forth slowly while the subject maintains visual fixation (eg, of the examiner's nose)

    b. The head impulse test: the head is moved quickly but not far

        i.   A catch-up saccade at the end of the head rotation indicates a poor VOR

        ii. The head impulse test has two advantages: it can test any single canal in isolation and it is less likely to be confounded by pursuit. The head impulse test is the best bedside test for impaired peripheral vestibular function

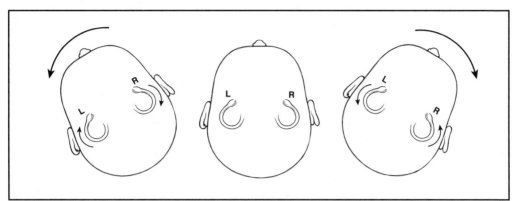

Figure 2-10. Doll's eye testing. When the head is rotated to the left, the endolymph moves toward the left ampulla and away from the right ampulla. When the head is rotated to the right, the endolymph moves toward the right ampulla and away from the left ampulla.

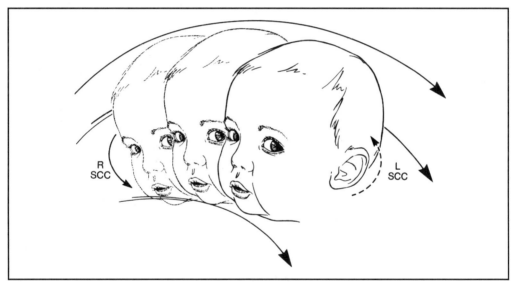

Figure 2-11. Rotational testing for eye movement function in infants. As the infant is turned toward his or her left (toward the examiner's right), the eye will tonically deviate in the direction of the movement with jerk phase of nystagmus toward the opposite side. This leads to stimulation of the right semicircular canals (SCC) and inhibition of the left SCC.

        c.   Head rotation testing is helpful in assessing the range of eye movements in infants (Figure 2-11)

   2.   Caloric testing

        a.   Test of horizontal canal (HC) function

        b.   Uses a combination of gravity and a thermal gradient across the labyrinth to cause cupular deflection

        c.   The subject is positioned so that the HCs are oriented vertically, to maximize the effect of gravity on the endolymph (about 30 degrees up from the supine position) (Figure 2-12A)

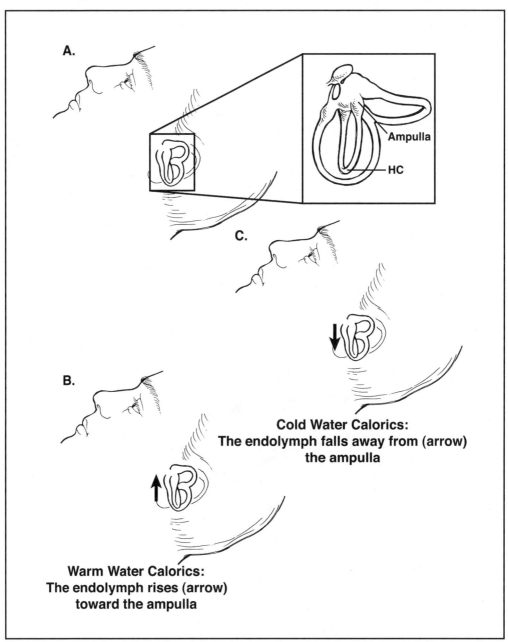

Figure 2-12. With head elevated 30 degrees, horizontal canal is oriented in vertical direction, allowing for maximal effect with caloric testing.

d.   The external auditory canal (EAC) is irrigated with warm (44°C) or cool (30°C) water (Figures 2-12B and 2-12C)

e.   Warm water is excitatory and cool water is inhibitory, eliciting a corresponding nystagmus

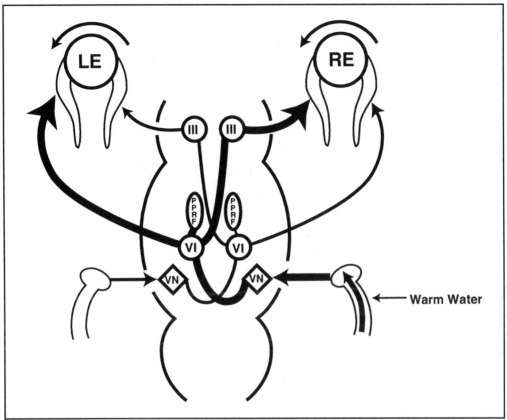

Figure 2-13. Warm water in the right ear causes shift of endolymph toward the ampulla, thereby increasing the vestibular tone and resulting in a slow movement of the eyes to the left side. The compensatory fast phase will be directed back to the right side.

       f.   Example: warm water in the right EAC excites the right HC, eliciting leftward slow phases and a right-beating nystagmus (Figure 2-13). Cool water inhibits the right HC and causes a left-beating nystagmus (Figure 2-14)

       g.   A lesion of one labyrinth will reduce the nystagmus from irrigation of that side

  3.   Comatose patients

       a.   Caloric irrigation is used to test whether the lower brainstem is intact in comatose patients

       b.   To maximize the stimulus, ice water is used

       c.   Comatose patients do not have quick phases, so there is no nystagmus, only a tonic drift of the eyes toward the irrigated (inhibited) ear

VI. Disorders of horizontal gaze

  A.   Cerebral cortical lesions

      1.   Acute cerebral hemisphere infarcts may cause conjugate eye deviation toward the lesion side

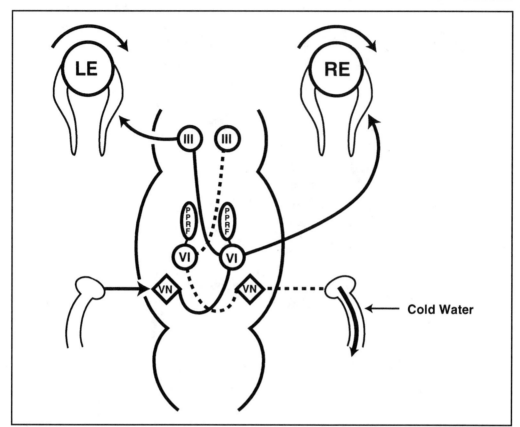

Figure 2-14. Cold water in the right ear causes shift of endolymph away from the ampulla, thereby decreasing the vestibular tone and allowing the vestibular tone from the left side to be dominant. This results in a slow movement of the eyes to the right. The compensatory fast phase will therefore be directed to the left side.

<ol type="a">
<li>Frontal and/or parietal ocular motor areas may be involved</li>
<li>Gaze deviation results from unopposed activity of the normal contralateral hemisphere and, with right hemisphere lesions, spatial neglect</li>
<li>Vestibular reflexes (VOR, calorics) remain intact and can still drive the eyes toward the contralateral side</li>
<li>Acute FEF lesions transiently impair contraversive saccades</li>
<li>Lesions of prefrontal cortex impair suppression of unwanted reflexive saccades</li>
</ol>

2. Congenital ocular motor apraxia

<ol type="a">
<li>Impairment of voluntary horizontal eye movements</li>
<li>Reflexive saccades and combined eye-head saccades (shifts of gaze with the head unrestrained) may be relatively spared</li>
<li>The VOR is normal</li>
<li>In more severe cases, quick phases may also be impaired</li>
<li>"Head thrusts" may be used to redirect gaze, when head-free saccades and vestibular quick phases are impaired</li>
</ol>

          i.   The head is rotated toward the target

          ii.   Without quick phases, the intact VOR moves the eyes to an extreme orbital position

          iii.   Further head rotation "drags" the eyes in the direction of the target

          iv.   Once the target is foveated, the head is rotated back, but gaze direction does not change, because the VOR is again active

      f.   Associated with: ataxia telangiectasia; ataxia with ocular motor apraxia, types 1 and 2; Joubert's syndrome; Niemann-Pick disease, type C; Gaucher's disease

   3.   Balint's syndrome

      a.   A form of acquired ocular motor apraxia due to bilateral posterior parietal lesions

      b.   Inability to shift gaze or attention to another location in the visual field

      c.   Simultanagnosia: inability to perceive more than one object at at time

      d.   The VOR is intact

      e.   Optic ataxia: impaired visually guided reaching

B.   Pontine lesions

   1.   Pontine conjugate gaze palsy

      a.   A lesion of the PPRF eliminates all ipsiversive saccades, due to loss of horizontal saccade burst neurons

      b.   If the abducens (CN VI) nucleus is involved, there will be a complete conjugate gaze palsy, affecting horizontal saccades, pursuit, optokinetic, and vestibular eye movements. The effect is conjugate because both abducens motoneurons and interneurons are lost

      c.   This gaze palsy distinguishes an abducens nucleus lesion from one affecting the abducens nerve, which only affects abduction of the ipsilateral eye

      d.   If only the PPRF (and not the abducens nucleus) is affected, the VOR is preserved

   2.   Internuclear ophthalmoplegia (INO)

      a.   A lesion of the MLF affects axons of contralateral abducens neurons that project to MR motoneurons of the ipsilateral oculomotor nucleus ("internuclear"=between nuclei VI and III)

      b.   Impaired adduction of the eye ipsilateral to the MLF lesion during attempted conjugate gaze away from the lesion (Figure 2-15)

      c.   There may be nystagmus of the abducting eye when looking away from the lesion

      d.   A complete INO eliminates adduction past the midline for all conjugate eye movements

      e.   A partial INO may only slow the adducting eye during contraversive saccades without affecting the overall range of adduction

      f.   The INO is named for the side of the lesion (a right INO impairs right eye adduction)

      g.   Usually adduction during convergence is relatively spared (Cogan posterior INO)

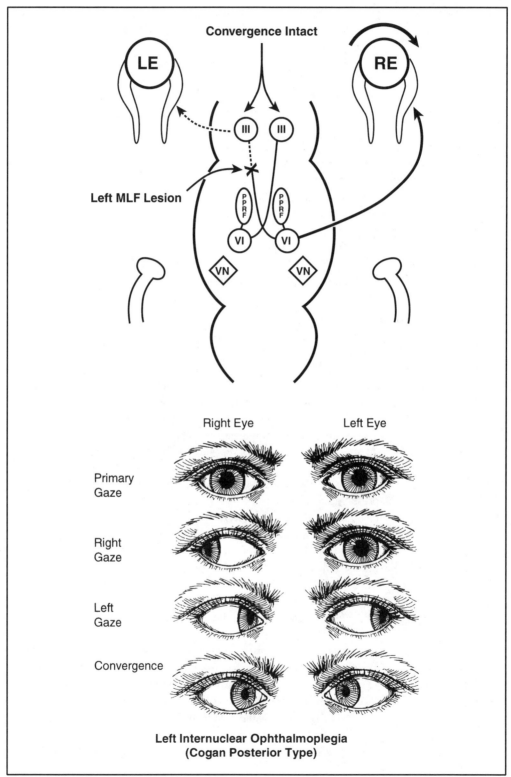

**Left Internuclear Ophthalmoplegia
(Cogan Posterior Type)**

Figure 2-15.

      h.   INO caused by a midbrain lesion may also affect convergence and is usually bilateral (Cogan anterior INO)

      i.   INO (unilateral or bilateral) in a young adult is most commonly due to multiple sclerosis; in adults over 50, ischemia is the most common cause

      j.   WEBINO (wall-eyed bilateral INO) refers to exotropia with bilateral INOs. It is impossible to exclude involvement of the MR subnuclei along with both MLFs, unless convergence is spared

      k.   INO may be accompanied by:

          i.   Skew deviation (hypertropia of the ipsilateral eye)/ocular tilt reaction

          ii.   Disjunctive vertical-torsional nystagmus

          iii.   Impaired VOR in response to head impulses exciting the contralateral posterior canal

   3.   One-and-a-half syndrome (Figure 2-16)

      a.   Caused by a unilateral pontine lesion that affects both the PPRF/abducens nucleus and the MLF

      b.   Conjugate ipsiversive gaze palsy ("one")

      c.   INO leading to impaired adduction of the ipsilateral eye during contraversive gaze (the "half")

      d.   For example, with a right one-and-a-half syndrome, neither eye can make rightward saccades and only the left eye can make leftward saccades

      e.   For the first few days, there may be an exotropia, due to tonic abduction of the contralateral eye (paralytic pontine exotropia)

VII. Disorders of vertical gaze

   A.   Downgaze palsy—due to midbrain disease (stroke, tumor) with lesions involving the riMLF just rostral to the oculomotor (CN III) nucleus and dorsomedial to the red nucleus. A unilateral riMLF lesion impairs downward (but not upward) saccades and ipsilesional torsional quick phases. The latter can be tested with head roll

   B.   Upgaze palsy—associated with lesions located more dorsally, including the posterior commissure

   C.   Vertical gaze palsies are occasionally monocular

   D.   riMLF control of upward saccades is bilateral but of downward saccades is unilateral at the OMN level. Each riMLF projects to the neurons innervating the ipsilateral inferior rectus and contralateral superior oblique. Thus, a unilateral riMLF lesion impairs downward (but not upward) saccades

   E.   The riMLF also generates torsional components of saccades and quick phases. A unilateral riMLF lesion impairs ipsilesional torsional quick phases (eg, a right riMLF lesion affects clockwise—from the patient's perspective—quick phases)

   F.   Dorsal midbrain syndrome

      1.   Also known as "pretectal syndrome," "Sylvian aqueduct syndrome," and "Parinaud's syndrome"

      2.   Supranuclear paresis of vertical gaze, especially upward, reflecting involvement of the INC and its projections through the posterior commissure

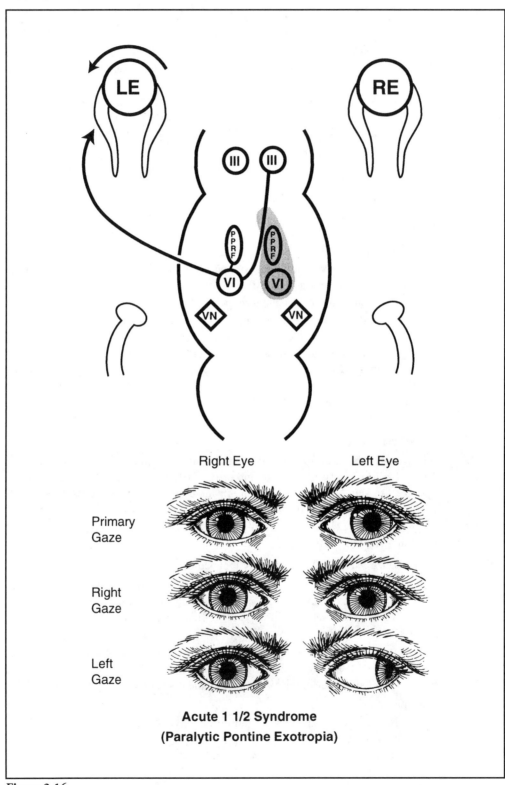

Acute 1 1/2 Syndrome
(Paralytic Pontine Exotropia)

Figure 2-16.

3. Other associated eye signs:
   a. Light-near dissociation of the pupils—pupils constrict with near viewing but not to light
   b. Convergence-retraction nystagmus
   c. Lid retraction (Collier's sign)
   d. Convergence spasm or paresis
   e. Accommodative spasm or paresis
   f. Skew deviation (see Chapter 2, IX)

G. Progressive supranuclear palsy (PSP)
   1. Supranuclear impairment of voluntary and reflexive saccades
   2. Vertical saccades (especially downward) are affected first, but horizontal saccades also become involved as the disease progresses
   3. First, saccade velocities are reduced, but eventually all gaze movements are lost
   4. Neck rigidity makes it difficult for patients to use head movements to shift gaze
   5. The VOR remains intact until very late in the disease course
   6. Other features:
      a. Strabismus
      b. Reduced blinking, leading to corneal drying
      c. Eyelid opening apraxia (slowed eye opening after eye closure)
      d. Gaze-evoked nystagmus
   7. Similar syndromes can occur due to central nervous system ischemia and after cardiac surgery

H. Oculogyric crisis
   1. Tonic, involuntary deviation of the eyes, usually upward, sometimes horizontal
   2. Associated with neuroleptics and other drugs, encephalitis lethargica (postencephalitic parkinsonism)

VIII. Disorders of vergence

A. Spasm of the near reflex
   1. Triad of convergence, accommodation, miosis
   2. May simulate unilateral or bilateral abducens palsies
   3. Usually psychogenic with a variable esotropia
   4. Rarely due to organic disease: head trauma, dorsal midbrain syndrome, intoxication, Wernicke's syndrome

B. Convergence paresis/paralysis
   1. Patients report diplopia at near or easy fatigability when reading
   2. Usual causes: aging, lack of effort
   3. Rarely due to organic cause: dorsal midbrain syndrome, multiple sclerosis, encephalitis, diphtheria, botulism

C. Divergence paresis/paralysis
   1. Characterized by:
      a. Orthophoria at near

        b.   Comitant esotropia at distance

        c.   Full extraocular movements

   2.   May present in isolation in adults without other neurologic findings

   3.   Must exclude:

        a.   Decompensated esophoria

        b.   Subtle bilateral abducens palsies

   4.   Causes: head trauma, PSP, brainstem stroke, cerebellar lesions including Arnold-Chiari I malformation

   5.   Esotropia when looking at distance is a characteristic finding in cerebellar disease (most likely due to involvement of the vermis)

IX.   Skew deviation

A.   Vertical/torsional strabismus from a supranuclear lesion

B.   Must be distinguished from a cyclovertical extraocular muscle palsy (eg, superior oblique palsy)

C.   Usually due to lesion in central otolith pathways or INC. May be part of a full ocular tilt reaction (see below) or may occur in isolation

D.   May be comitant or incomitant

E.   Sometimes associated with internuclear ophthalmoplegia (MLF lesion) or vertical/ torsional nystagmus

F.   With lower brainstem lesions, the ipsilateral eye is usually hypotropic; with pontine and midbrain lesions, the ipsilateral eye is usually hypertropic

G.   An alternating skew deviation is a characteristic finding in cerebellar degeneration; usually the abducting eye is higher

X.   Ocular tilt reaction

A.   Caused by a lesion in the peripheral or central otolith pathways that carry signals from the utricle

B.   Normally the utricle is excited by ipsilateral head tilt and inhibited by contralateral head tilt

C.   Physiologic ocular tilt reaction: the normal response to head tilt is to move the head back toward upright, to counterroll the eyes, and (in lateral-eyed animals) to produce a vertical vergence movement to realign both eyes with the horizontal

D.   If one utricle is lesioned, the tonic signal from the other side is unopposed, leading to an input imbalance, as if the head were tilted toward the good side

E.   Pathologic ocular tilt reaction (Figure 2-17)

   1.   Head tilt toward the lesioned ear (because the brain thinks the head is tilted toward the good side and wants to restore it to upright)

   2.   Ocular rotation (torsion), with the upper poles of the eyes moving toward the lesioned side (the appropriate ocular counterroll if the head were tilted toward the good side, as the brain thinks)

   3.   Skew deviation: disconjugate vertical deviation with the eye on the lesioned side lower (the appropriate response in a lateral-eyed animal, if the head were tilted toward the good side)

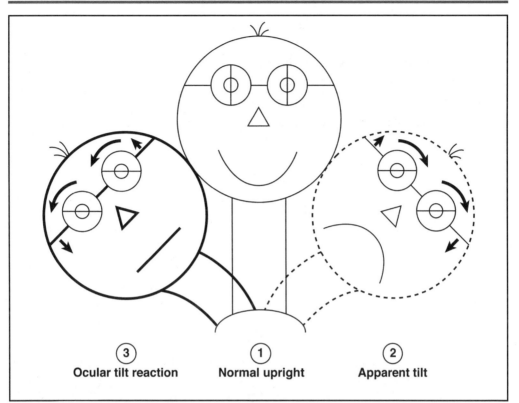

Figure 2-17. With the ocular tilt reaction, apparent tilt of the environment (2) is compensated for (3) to achieve appearance of normal upright orientation (1). With ocular tilt reaction the upper poles of each eye rotate toward the lower ear. (Modified from Brandt T, Dieterich M. Pathological eye-hand coordination in roll: tonic ocular tilt reaction in mesencephalic and medullary lesions. *Brain.* 1987;110:649-666.)

    F.   Utricular afferents synapse in the vestibular nuclei, whose neurons project across the midline into the contralateral MLF. Thus, an MLF lesion produces a contraversive ocular tilt reaction (the head tilts and the eyes rotate away from the side of the MLF lesion and the ipsilateral eye is higher)

XI.   Wernicke's encephalopathy

    A.   Critical to recognize because it must be treated promptly

    B.   Triad: ophthalmoplegia, mental confusion, gait ataxia

    C.   Caused by thiamine deficiency (alcoholism, malnutrition)

    D.   Ocular motor findings include:

        1.   Impaired abduction

        2.   Partial or complete ophthalmoplegia

        3.   Vertical nystagmus, usually upbeat, that may change direction with convergence

        4.   Vestibular hypofunction

5.   Gaze-evoked nystagmus

6.   Internuclear ophthalmoplegia

E.   Lesions occur throughout the brainstem, thalamus, hypothalamus, cerebellum

F.   Treated emergently with intravenous thiamine

G.   Magnesium deficiency must be tested for and treated if present

H.   If untreated, may progress to Korsakoff's syndrome with permanent memory loss and persistent eye movement abnormalities

BIBLIOGRAPHY

Books

Leigh RJ, Zee DS. *The Neurology of Eye Movements*. 4th ed. New York, NY: Oxford University Press; 2006.

Chapters

Buttner–Ennever JA, ed. Neuroanatomy of the oculomotor system. *Progress in Brain Research*. Vol 151. New York, NY: Elsevier; 2006.

Buttner U, Brandt T. Ocular motor disorders of the brainstem. In: Buttner U, Brandt T. *Balliere's Clinical Neurology*. Philadelphia, Pa: Balliere Tindoll; 1992.

Lavin PJM, Donahue SP. Neuro-ophthalmology: ocular motor system. In: Bradley WG, Daroff RB, Fenichel GM, Jankovic J, eds. *Neurology in Clinical Practice*. 4th ed. Boston, Mass: Butterworth-Heineman; 2003:chap 39.

Leigh RJ, Daroff RB, Troost BT. Supranuclear disorders of eye movements. In: Glaser JS, ed. *Neuro-Ophthalmology*. 3rd ed. Philadelphia, Pa: Lippincott Williams & Wilkins; 1999:345-368.

Sharpe J, Wong AMF. Anatomy and physiology of ocular motor systems. In: Miller NR, Newman NJ, eds. *Walsh and Hoyt's Clinical Neuro-Ophthalmology*. 6th ed. Vol 1. Philadelphia, Pa: Lippincott Williams & Wilkins; 2005:809-885.

Zee DS, Newman-Toker DE. Supranuclear and internuclear ocular motility disorders. In: Miller NR, Newman NJ, eds. *Walsh and Hoyt's Clinical Neuro-Ophthalmology*. 6th ed. Vol 1. Philadelphia, Pa: Lippincott Williams & Wilkins; 2005:907-967.

Articles

Baker RS, Epstein AD. Ocular motor abnormalities from head trauma. *Surv Ophthalmol*. 1991;35:245-267.

Bhidayasiri R, Plant GT, Leigh RJ. A hypothetical scheme for the brainstem control of vertical gaze. *Neurology*. 2000;54:1985-1993.

Brandt T, Dieterich M. Vestibular syndromes in the roll plane: topographic diagnosis from brainstem to cortex. *Ann Neurol*. 1994;36:337-347.

Brodsky MC, Donahue SP, Vaphiades M, Brandt T. Skew deviation revisited. *Surv Ophthalmol*. 2006;51:105-128.

Cogan DG. Congenital ocular motor apraxia. *Can J Ophthalmol*. 1966;1:253-260.

Donahue SP, Lavin PJ, Hamed LM. Tonic ocular tilt reaction simulating a superior oblique palsy. Diagnostic confusion with the three-step test. *Arch Ophthalmol*. 1999;117:347-352.

Fisher CM. Some neuro-ophthalmological observations. *J Neurol Neurosurg Psychiatry.* 1967;30:383-392.

Halmagyi GM, Curthoys IS. A clinical sign of canal paresis. *Arch Neurol.* 1988;45:737-739.

Krauzlis RJ. Recasting the smooth pursuit eye movement system. *J Neurophysiol.* 2004;91:591-603.

Ramat S, Leigh RJ, Zee DS, Optican LM. What clinical disorders tell us about the neural control of saccadic eye movements. *Brain.* 2007;130:10-35.

Chapter 3

Nystagmus and Related Ocular Oscillations

Mark F. Walker, MD, and Lanning B. Kline, MD

I. **Nystagmus is a rhythmic, involuntary, back-and-forth oscillation of the eyes**

    A. Nystagmus is categorized by its waveform (Figure 3-1)

        1. Jerk (most common): slow drift (slow phase) followed by quick reset (quick phase). Slow phase waveform can be:

            a. Increasing velocity exponential (eg, integrator instability, congenital)

            b. Decreasing velocity exponential (eg, gaze-evoked)

            c. Constant (linear) velocity (eg, vestibular)

        2. Pendular: sinusoidal oscillation (like a pendulum), phases have equal speed

    B. Trajectory: nystagmus can be horizontal, vertical, torsional, or a combination of the three

        1. Combined horizontal and vertical pendular nystagmus can be diagonal or elliptical, depending on the difference in phase between the two components

        2. Seesaw nystagmus: alternating upward/excyclotorsional movement of one eye with downward/incyclotorsional movement of the other eye (hemiseesaw: one direction is a quick phase)

    C. The direction of jerk nystagmus is usually defined by its quick phases ("right-beating nystagmus": eyes drift left and beat right)

    D. Conjugacy: nystagmus can be conjugate (both eyes move in the same direction) or disconjugate (the eyes move in different directions, also called disjunctive)

    E. Dissociated: the two eyes move in the same direction but by different amounts

    F. Alexander's law: jerk nystagmus usually increases in intensity when looking in the direction of the quick phase

    G. Null zone: the field of gaze where nystagmus intensity is minimal

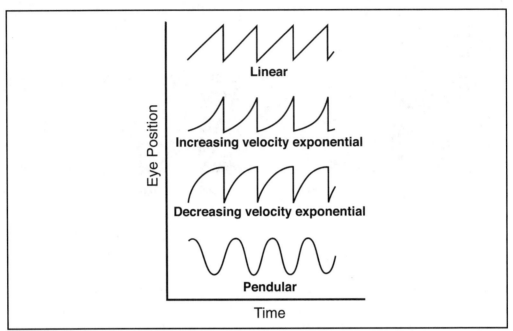

Figure 3-1. Nystagmus waveforms named for the velocity profile of the slow phase. Linear is typical of vestibular nystagmus, increasing velocity exponential of congenital nystagmus, decreasing velocity exponential of gaze-evoked nystagmus, and pendular may be seen with congenital or acquired nystagmus.

II. **Physiologic nystagmus (not all nystagmus is pathological)**

    A.   End-position nystagmus: a few beats of horizontal nystagmus when the eyes are first moved to extreme horizontal positions in the orbit

    B.   Vestibular nystagmus (see Chapter 2)

        1.   Caloric nystagmus

            a.   Irrigation with warm water (in the head-up supine position) causes endolymph in the horizontal canal to move toward the ampulla, exciting the hair cells and driving a slow phase eye movement away from the irrigated side

            b.   Irrigation with cold water inhibits the horizontal canal and produces a slow phase toward the irrigated side

        2.   Rotational nystagmus (vestibulo-ocular reflex [VOR])

            a.   Prolonged head rotation produces a slow phase in the direction opposite to head movement interrupted by quick phases in the same direction as head movement

            b.   This serves to stabilize the retinal image as the head moves

    C.   Optokinetic nystagmus (OKN)

        1.   Driven by prolonged full-field visual motion

        2.   In natural circumstances, most often occurs during sustained self-rotation in the light

        3.   Supplements the VOR to stabilize vision

III. Pathologic nystagmus

    A.   Congenital nystagmus (infantile nystagmus syndrome)

        1.   May be present at birth but more commonly appears later in infancy

        2.   May be sporadic or genetic

            a.   Autosomal dominant (6p12), autosomal recessive, and X-linked recessive patterns seen

            b.   Associated with oculocutaneous albinism

        3.   Commonly accentuated by attempted fixation and anxiety

        4.   Typically damped by eye closure and convergence

        5.   May or may not be accompanied by abnormalities of the visual system

        6.   Does not cause oscillopsia

        7.   Distinct waveforms

            a.   Usually conjugate horizontal-torsional pendular and/or jerk nystagmus

            b.   Similar amplitude in both eyes

            c.   Jerk nystagmus has increasing velocity slow phases

            d.   Foveation periods: brief cessation of eye motion, often following quick phases, during which clear vision is possible (if there are no afferent visual abnormalities)

        8.   There is often an orbital position (null point) where nystagmus is minimal and vision is best

        9.   May be associated with other abnormalities: strabismus, latent nystagmus, head oscillations

    B.   Latent nystagmus (fusional maldevelopment nystagmus syndrome)

        1.   Seen only when one eye is covered

        2.   Binocular jerk nystagmus with slow phases directed toward the covered eye

        3.   Linear or exponentially decreasing slow phase velocity profile

        4.   Retinal slip from nystagmus causes visual acuity to be diminished during monocular viewing

        5.   Binocular viewing suppresses nystagmus and improves visual acuity

        6.   May occur in association with congenital pendular or jerk nystagmus

        7.   May be associated with dissociated vertical deviation and strabismus (usually esotropia)

    C.   Manifest latent nystagmus

        1.   Similar to latent nystagmus but present with both eyes uncovered

        2.   Suppression of vision in one eye (eg, due to strabismus and amblyopia) is the functional equivalent of covering one eye

        3.   Slow phases directed away from the viewing eye (as in latent nystagmus)

        4.   Vision may be improved when the eyes are moved eccentrically in the orbits in the direction of the slow phase

    D.   Spasmus nutans

        1.   Triad of head turn, head nodding, and nystagmus

        2.   Typically develops during the first year of life

        3.   Resolves by age 10

        4.   Horizontal or vertical pendular nystagmus with low amplitude and high frequency

     5.   May be monocular or of different amplitude and/or phase in each eye

     6.   Optic pathway glioma can cause acquired monocular nystagmus and should be ruled out by magnetic resonance imaging

  E.   Seesaw nystagmus

     1.   A disconjugate vertical-torsional nystagmus

     2.   The torsional component has the same direction in both eyes but the vertical movement is in the opposite direction

     3.   During each half cycle, one eye moves upward and intorts and the other eye moves downward and extorts

     4.   May be pendular (seesaw nystagmus) or jerk (hemi-seesaw nystagmus)

     5.   Associated with:

        a.   Midbrain stroke

        b.   Medial medullary stroke

        c.   Multiple sclerosis

        d.   Chiari malformation

        e.   Head trauma

        f.   Visual loss

        g.   Parasellar masses

        h.   Congenital

  F.   Convergence-retraction nystagmus

     1.   Convergence and/or retraction of the eyes elicited by attempted upward saccades or quick phases

     2.   Best seen during stimulation with a downward-moving OKN stimulus

     3.   Part of the dorsal midbrain syndrome

        a.   Impaired vertical gaze (particularly upward)

        b.   Light-near dissociation of the pupillary responses

        c.   Lid retraction (Collier's sign)

        d.   Covergence-retraction nystagmus

        e.   Spasm or paresis of convergence

        f.   Spasm or paresis of accommodation

        g.   Skew deviation

     4.   Due to lesions affecting the area of the posterior commissure

        a.   Tumors (eg, pineal)

        b.   Hydrocephalus (eg, aqueductal stenosis)

        c.   Hemorrhage or infarction (midbrain, thalamus)

        d.   Multiple sclerosis and other inflammatory lesions

  G.   Downbeat nystagmus

     1.   Spontaneous upward drift of the eyes

     2.   Characteristic sign of a lesion of the vestibulocerebellum or its pathways in the brainstem (cerebellar degeneration, multiple sclerosis, stroke)

     3.   Other important causes include drug toxicity (lithium, anticonvulsants), Wernicke's encephalopathy

     4.   Often occurs in the context of a more general cerebellar syndrome but may present in isolation and be nonprogressive

     5.   Slow phase waveform may have constant, decreasing, or increasing velocity

     6.   Commonly enhanced by down and lateral gaze

     7.   May be affected by vergence state, position of the head relative to gravity (eg, prone vs supine positioning)

H.   Upbeat nystagmus

     1.   Spontaneous nystagmus with downward slow phases in primary position

     2.   Different from upbeat nystagmus that may be a part of gaze-evoked nystagmus and is only present when looking up (not in primary position) and also from the transient upbeat nystagmus seen in benign paroxysmal positioning vertigo (BPPV) (see below)

     3.   Etiologies:

          a.   Focal lesions (infarction, tumor, demyelinating) of the medulla or cerebellum

          b.   Cerebellar degeneration

          c.   Wernicke's encephalopathy

     4.   Downbeat nystagmus may convert to upbeat nystagmus with convergence (or vice versa)

I.   Gaze-evoked and rebound nystagmus

     1.   Loss of eccentric gaze holding, in which the eyes tend to drift back to the center of the orbit

     2.   A weak neural integrator does not produce a sufficiently strong tonic innervation to hold the eyes against elastic forces

     3.   Etiologies

          a.   Vestibulocerebellar lesions (eg, cerebellar degenerations)

          b.   Functional neural integrator impairment due to drugs (sedatives, anticonvulsants), metabolic derangements

     4.   The direction of nystagmus depends on gaze direction: the eyes drift toward the center and quick phases beat back in the direction of attempted gaze

     5.   Typically horizontal: right-beating nystagmus with right gaze and left-beating nystagmus with left gaze

     6.   May also include upbeat nystagmus with upgaze

     7.   With sustained gaze, the nystagmus will often diminish

     8.   Upon return to center position, there may be a brief oppositely directed nystagmus (rebound nystagmus)

     9.   Gaze-evoked and downbeat nystagmus often occur together in patients with cerebellar degeneration

J.   Pendular nystagmus

     1.   Sinusoidal oscillation (no quick phases)

     2.   May have a complex waveform that includes horizontal, vertical, and torsional components

     3.   Elliptical nystagmus: horizontal and vertical components out of phase

     4.   May be congenital (see above) or acquired

     5.   Etiologies of acquired pendular nystagmus

          a.   Multiple sclerosis

          b.   Oculopalatal tremor syndrome

          i.   Usually vertical-pendular nystagmus

          ii.   Synchronous contraction of face, palate, pharynx, diaphragm, extremities

          iii. Persist during sleep

          iv. Lesion: within "triangle of Guillain and Mollaret" connecting red nucleus, ipsilateral inferior olive, contralateral dentate nucleus

          v.   Seen with hypertrophy of inferior olive (latency from acute infarction: 2 to 49 months); not a manifestation of an acute lesion

     c.   Whipple's disease

     d.   Pelizaeus-Merzbacher disease

     e.   Toluene toxicity

     f.   Severe visual loss

  6.   May respond to gabapentin or memantine

K.   Periodic alternating nystagmus (PAN)

  1.   Horizontal jerk nystagmus that changes direction every 2 minutes

  2.   Present in the primary position, unlike gaze-evoked nystagmus

  3.   May be accompanied by periodic head deviations that reduce the nystagmus by moving the eyes into a relative null position

  4.   Results from lesions to the vestibulocerebellum (nodulus/uvula) combined with either flocculus/paraflocculus lesions or visual loss

  5.   Baclofen abolishes nystagmus

  6.   In cases where visual loss contributes, improvement of vision (eg, vitrectomy, cataract extraction) may eliminate nystagmus

  7.   Congenital PAN is less regularly periodic than acquired PAN and does not respond as well to baclofen

  8.   In comatose patients with no quick phases, PAN may be seen as a periodic alternating gaze deviation

L.   Peripheral vestibular nystagmus

  1.   Jerk nystagmus due to imbalance of vestibular inputs (see Chapter 2)

  2.   Unilateral vestibular hypofunction

     a.   An acute lesion to one labyrinth or vestibular nerve (eg, vestibular neuritis) results in a spontaneous horizontal/torsional nystagmus, because the tonic input from the intact side is suddenly unopposed

     b.   The eyes drift (slow phase) toward the lesioned side and quick phases beat toward the intact side

     c.   The intensity is usually greatest when looking toward the intact side (Alexander's law), but the direction does not change with gaze, unlike gaze-evoked nystagmus

     d.   May be partially or fully suppressed by vision and is best seen when fixation is removed

          i.   Frenzel goggles

          ii.   When looking at one optic nerve with a direct ophthalmoscope, cover the fellow eye

     e.   Slowly growing tumors (eg, vestibular schwannomas) do not usually produce much nystagmus because the vestibular imbalance is compensated centrally as it develops (may see Bruns' nystagmus—see next page)

        f.   Bilateral vestibular lesions do not cause nystagmus because the lesion is symmetric and there is no imbalance

   3.   Bruns' nystagmus

        a.   May be seen with large tumors in the cerebellopontine angle

        b.   Two components:

            i.   Horizontal nystagmus beating away from the lesion when looking away from the lesion (vestibular nystagmus—accentuated by Alexander's law) due to vestibular nerve involvement

           ii.   Horizontal nystagmus beating toward the lesion when looking toward the lesion (unilateral gaze-evoked nystagmus) due to compression of the adjacent brainstem and cerebellar flocculus

   4.   Benign paroxysmal positional nystagmus (BPPV)

        a.   Brief (<1 min) nystagmus provoked by changes in head position relative to gravity (lying down, looking up, rolling over in bed)

        b.   Caused by free-moving otoconia that have become lodged in a semicircular canal

        c.   Usually affects the posterior canal: slow phases are directed downward with a torsional component in which the upper poles of the eyes rotate away from the affected ear (upbeating-torsional nystagmus)

        d.   Diagnosed by the Dix-Hallpike maneuver

        e.   Treated by repositioning maneuvers (eg, Epley, Semont) that move the otoconia out of the affected canal

   5.   Sound (Tullio phenomenon) and pressure-induced nystagmus

        a.   Loud noise or pressure in the external ear causes endolymph motion due to the presence of a fistula

        b.   Usually caused by superior semicircular canal dehiscence (defect in the bony roof of the superior canal leading to a communication between the labyrinth and the middle cranial fossa)

        c.   If severe, treated surgically by closing the fistula

IV.   Saccadic intrusions and oscillations

   A.   Saccadic intrusions are undesired, involuntary saccades that interfere with visual fixation

   B.   Repeated saccadic intrusions result in saccadic oscillations

   C.   Saccadic oscillations differ from nystagmus in that they are made up only of saccades; there are no slow phases

   D.   Saccadic oscillations are defined by their amplitude, frequency, direction, and whether they have a normal intersaccadic interval

   E.   Square-wave jerks and square-wave oscillations

        1.   A square-wave jerk consists of an involuntary saccade (amplitude 0.5 to 3 degrees) followed by a second saccade after a normal interval (about 200 msec) that brings the eyes back to the point of fixation

        2.   Square-wave jerks may be seen in normal individuals but are enhanced in neurological diseases such as cerebellar lesions and progressive supranuclear palsy

        3.   Named for their rectangular appearance on eye movement recordings

    4.   Macro-square-wave jerks are larger (>5 degrees) and have a shorter intersaccadic interval

    5.   Macrosaccadic oscillations are repeated saccades with a normal intersaccadic interval that are related to saccadic hypermetria and usually seen with lesions of the cerebellar vermis

F.   Ocular flutter and opsoclonus

    1.   Continuous back-to-back saccades without an intersaccadic interval

    2.   Symptoms are blurred vision and oscillopsia

    3.   May be associated with limb and body myoclonus

    4.   Ocular flutter is a one-dimensional (usually horizontal) saccadic oscillation; opsoclonus has horizontal, vertical, and torsional components

    5.   Causes:

        a.   Para-infectious encephalitis of the brainstem

        b.   Paraneoplastic syndrome

        c.   Toxic-metabolic

        d.   Idiopathic

    6.   The opsoclonus-myoclonus syndrome in children is characteristic of a neuroblastoma

    7.   In adults other tumors (breast, small-cell lung, ovary) are associated with paraneoplastic flutter and opsoclonus

    8.   Treatment includes removing the tumor, if present. Immune therapies, such as IV Ig, may help

G.   Microsaccadic oscillations (microflutter)

    1.   Very small amplitude flutter

    2.   Usually requires an ophthalmoscope to visualize

    3.   May be isolated and benign, but evaluation for an occult malignancy should be performed

    4.   Can be multidirectional: microsaccadic opsoclonus

H.   Voluntary flutter (voluntary "nystagmus")

    1.   Saccadic oscillation (not true nystagmus) that can be induced, often by vergence effort

    2.   Unlike involuntary flutter and opsoclonus, it is not sustained

    3.   May produce oscillopsia when present

V.   Ocular bobbing variants and ping-pong gaze

A.   Ocular bobbing and its variants are vertical nystagmoid movements that occur in comatose patients

B.   Ocular bobbing is typically seen with pontine lesions (eg, hemorrhage or compression) but may occur with toxic-metabolic insults; the other variants are less well localized

C.   Ocular bobbing variants are distinguished by the pattern of slow and fast eye motion

    1.   Ocular bobbing: rapid downward movement followed by slow upward drift back to the center of the orbit

    2.   Reverse ocular bobbing: rapid upward movement followed by slow downward drift to center position

3. Ocular dipping (inverse ocular bobbing): slow downward drift with rapid upward return to center position
4. Reverse ocular dipping (converse ocular bobbing): slow upward drift followed by rapid downward return to center position

D. Ping-pong gaze is an alternating horizontal gaze deviation (changes every few seconds) that is seen in comatose patients

BIBLIOGRAPHY

Books

Leigh RJ, Zee DS. *The Neurology of Eye Movements*. 4th ed. New York, NY: Oxford University Press; 2006.

Chapters

Burde RM, Savino PJ, Trobe JD. *Clinical Decisions in Neuro-Ophthalmology*. 3rd ed. St Louis, Mo: CV Mosby; 2002:220-245.

Dell'Osso LF, Daroff RB. Nystagmus and saccadic intrusions and oscillations. In: Glaser JS. *Neuro-Ophthalmology*. 3rd ed. Philadelphia, Pa: Lippincott Williams & Wilkins; 1999:369-401.

Lavin PJM. Eye movement disorders: diplopia, mystagmus, and other ocular oscillations. In: Bradley WG, Daroff RB, Fenichel GM, Jankovic J, eds. *Neurology in Clinical Practice*. 4th ed. Boston, Mass: Butterworth-Heineman; 2003:chap 16.

Leigh RJ, Rucker JC. Nystagmus and related motility disorders. In: Miller NR, Newman NJ, eds. *Walsh and Hoyt's Clinical Neuro-Ophthalmology*. 6th ed. Vol 1. Philadelphia, Pa: Lippincott Williams & Wilkins; 2005:1133-1173.

Articles

Averbach-Heller L, Tusa RJ, Fuhry L, et al. A double-blind study of gabapentin and baclofen as treatment for acquired nystagmus. *Ann Neurol*. 1997;41:818-825.

Brandt S, Carlsen N, Glentin P, et al. Encephalopathia myoclonica infantalis (Kinsbourne) and neuroblastoma in children. A report of three cases. *Dev Med Child Neurol*. 1974;16:286-294.

Brazis PW. Ocular motor abnormalities in Wallenberg's lateral medullary syndrome. *Mayo Clin Proc*. 1992;67:365-378.

Cogan DG. Downbeat nystagmus. *Arch Ophthalmol*. 1968;80:757-768.

Gottlob I, Wizov SS, Reinecke RD, et al. Spasmus nutans. A long term follow-up. *Invest Ophthalmol Vis Sci*. 1995;36:2768-2771.

Hirose G, Kawada J, Tsukada K, et al. Upbeat nystagmus: clinicopathological and pathophysiological considerations. *J Neurol Sci*. 1991;105:159-167.

Kerrison JB, Arnould VJ, Barnada MM, et al. A gene for autosomal dominant congenital nystagmus localizes to 6p12. *Genomics*. 1996;33:523-526.

Lopez LI, Gresty MA, Bronstein AM, et al. Acquired pendular nystagmus; oculomotor and MRI findings. *Brain*. 1996;119:265-272.

McLean R, Proudlock F, Thomas S, Degg C, Gottlob I. Congenital nystagmus: randomized, controlled, double-masked trial of memantine/gabapentin. *Ann Neurol*. 2007;61:130-138.

Ramat S, Leigh RJ, Zee DS, Optican LM. What clinical disorders tell us about the neural control of saccadic eye movements. *Brain*. 2007;130:10-35.

Self J, Lotery A. The molecular genetics of congenital idiopathic nystagmus. *Semin Ophthalmol.* 2006;21:87-90.

Straube A. Therapeutic considerations for eye movement disorders. *Dev Ophthalmol.* 2007;40:175-192.

Strupp M, Brandt T. Pharmacological advances in the treatment of neuro-otological and eye movement disorders. *Curr Opin Neurol.* 2006;19:33-40.

Chapter 4

The Six Syndromes of the VI Nerve (Abducens)

Lanning B. Kline, MD

I. **Anatomical considerations**

   A.   Figures 4-1a and 4-1b identify the structures in the posterior fossa, base of the skull, and middle cranial fossa that serve as landmarks in the study of the VI nerve

   B.   Figure 4-2 is a schematic representation of these structures and includes a sagittal section of the brainstem

   C.   Figure 4-3 is a schematic representation of these structures when viewed from the occipital pole

   D.   Figure 4-4 illustrates the S-shaped course of the VI nerve and shows its relationship to the VII and VIII cranial nerves and the internal carotid artery

   E.   Figure 4-5 adds the III, IV, and V cranial nerves

   F.   Figure 4-6 shows the composite diagram and the division of the course of the VI nerve into five portions, each associated with a different syndrome:
   1. VI_1: the brainstem syndrome
   2. VI_2: the subarachnoid space syndrome
   3. VI_3: the petrous apex syndrome
   4. VI_4: the cavernous sinus syndrome
   5. VI_5: the orbital syndrome

II. **The brainstem syndrome (VI_1)**

   A.   Figure 4-6 reminds us that a brainstem lesion of the VI nerve may also affect V, VII, VIII nerves and the cerebellum

   B.   The VI nerve nucleus contains motoneurons that supply the lateral rectus muscle and abducens internuclear neurons that project via the medial longitudinal fasciculus (MLF) to the medial rectus subdivision of the contralateral oculomotor nucleus. Thus, a nuclear VI nerve palsy causes an ipsilateral conjugate horizontal gaze palsy

   C.   Figure 4-7 illustrates the structures within the substance of the lower pons that may be affected by a lesion affecting the VI nerve

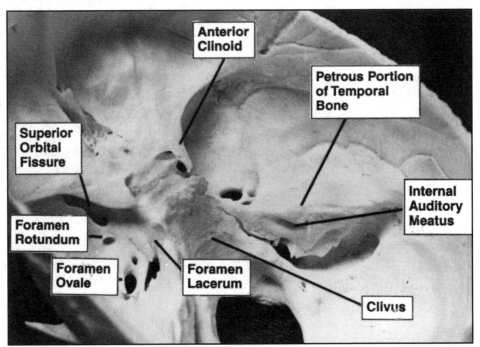

Figure 4-1a. Human skull. Anatomical landmarks in the study of the VI nerve. Oblique superotemporal view.

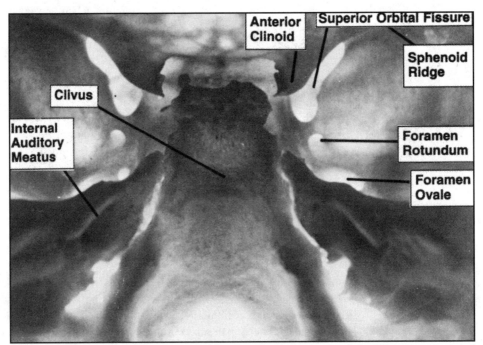

Figure 4-1b. Human skull. Anatomical landmarks in the study of the VI nerve. Occipital view, retroilluminated skull.

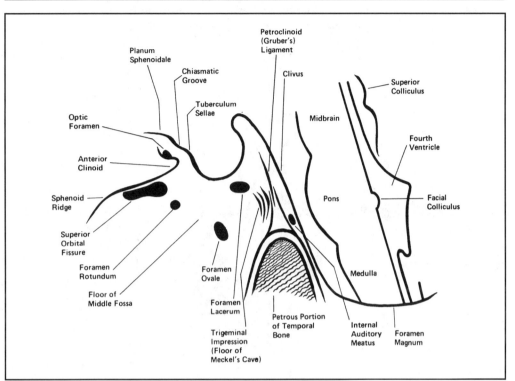

Figure 4-2. Schematic representation of the landmarks, temporal view.

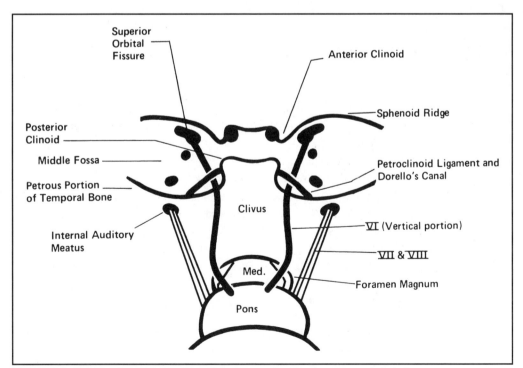

Figure 4-3. Schematic representation of the anatomical landmarks, occipital view.

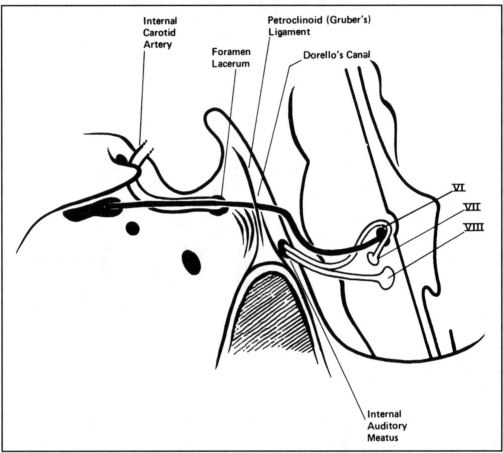

Figure 4-4. Course of the VI nerve (highlighted in black) from the pons to the superior orbital tissue.

       1. Oculosympathetic central neuron: ipsilateral Horner's syndrome

       2. Paramedian pontine reticular formation (PPRF): ipsilateral horizontal conjugate gaze palsy

       3. MLF: ipsilateral internuclear ophthalmoplegia

       4. Pyramidal tract: contralateral hemiparesis

   D. The brainstem syndrome may consist of any combination of the deficits listed above; the following are frequently encountered syndromes:

       1. Millard-Gubler syndrome

          a. VI nerve paresis

          b. Ipsilateral VII nerve paresis

          c. Contralateral hemiparesis

       2. Raymond's syndrome

          a. VI nerve paresis

          b. Contralateral hemiparesis

       3. Foville's syndrome

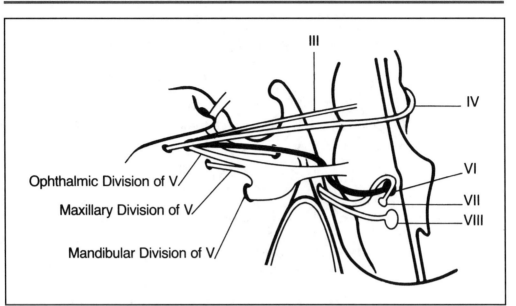

Figure 4-5. Composite diagram illustrating the III through VIII cranial nerves.

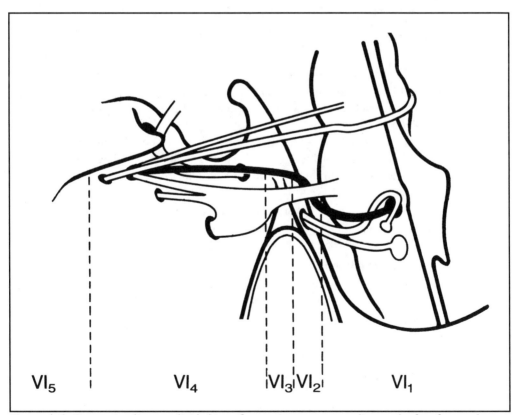

Figure 4-6. Composite diagram divided into five sections, corresponding to the first five syndromes of the VI nerve (VI_1 to VI_5).

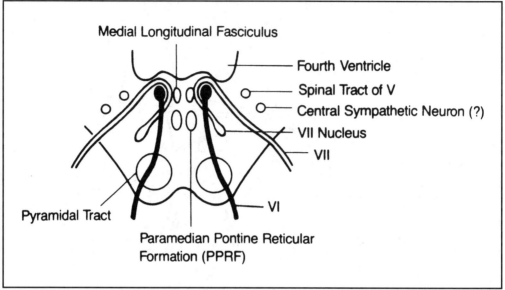

Figure 4-7. Diagram of cross-section of the lower pons through the VI nucleus and fascicle (highlighted in black).

      a.   Horizontal conjugate gaze palsy

      b.   Ipsilateral V, VII, VIII cranial nerve palsies

      c.   Ipsilateral Horner's syndrome

III.   The subarachnoid space syndrome (VI$_2$)

    A.   Elevated intracranial pressure may result in downward displacement of the brainstem, with stretching of the VI nerve, which is tethered at its exit from the pons and in Dorello's canal

       1.   Gives rise to "nonlocalizing" VI nerve palsies of raised intracranial pressure

       2.   Approximately 30% of patients with pseudotumor cerebri have VI nerve paresis, the only neurologic deficit they are allowed, besides papilledema and its visual field changes

    B.   Other disturbances in the subarachnoid space causing VI nerve palsies include hemorrhage, meningeal or parameningeal infection (eg, viral, bacterial, fungal), inflammation (eg, sarcoidosis), or infiltration (eg, lymphoma, leukemia, carcinoma)

IV.   The petrous apex syndrome (VI$_3$)

    A.   Contact with the tip of the petrous pyramid makes the portion of the VI nerve within Dorello's canal susceptible to pathologic processes affecting the petrous bone

    B.   Gradenigo's syndrome

       1.   Clinical findings

          a.   VI nerve palsy

          b.   Ipsilateral decreased hearing

          c.   Ipsilateral facial pain in the distribution of the V nerve

          d.   Ipsilateral facial paralysis

      2.   Due to localized inflammation or extradural abscess of petrous apex following complicated otitis media

   C.   Petrous bone fracture

      1.   Basal skull fracture following head trauma

      2.   Potential cranial nerve involvement: V, VI, VII, VIII

      3.   Associated findings: hemotympanum, Battle's sign, mastoid ecchymosis, cerebrospinal fluid otorrhea

   D.   Pseudo-Gradenigo's syndrome

      1.   Nasopharyngeal carcinoma: may cause serous otitis media due to obstruction of the eustachian tube and the carcinoma may subsequently invade the cavernous sinus, causing VI nerve paresis

      2.   Cerebellopontine angle tumor: may cause VI nerve paresis and other clinical findings, including:

         a.   Decreased hearing

         b.   VII nerve palsy

         c.   V nerve paralysis

         d.   Ataxia

         e.   Papilledema

V.   The cavernous sinus syndrome (VI_4)

   A.   Lesions in cavernous sinus rarely produce isolated VI nerve palsy; associated involvement of:

      1.   III, IV, and ophthalmic (V_1) nerves

      2.   Carotid oculosympathetic plexus (Horner's syndrome)

      3.   Optic nerve and chiasm

      4.   Pituitary gland

   B.   Differential diagnosis of cavernous sinus disease includes:

      1.   Trauma

      2.   Vascular

      3.   Neoplastic

      4.   Inflammatory

   C.   See Chapter 7

VI.   The orbital syndrome (VI_5)

   A.   Proptosis is an early sign and may be accompanied by congestion of the conjunctival vessels and chemosis

   B.   The optic nerve may appear normal or demonstrate atrophy or edema

   C.   Trigeminal signs are limited to the ophthalmic division

   D.   It is frequently difficult to distinguish between cranial nerve (III, IV, VI) pareses and mechanical restriction of the globe

   E.   Etiologies

      1.   Tumor (local, metastatic)

      2.   Trauma

      3.   Nonspecific orbital inflammation (pseudotumor)

      4.   Cellulitis

VII. Isolated VI nerve palsy (VI$_6$)

    A.   The sixth syndrome of the VI nerve

        1.   No signs of the first five syndromes

        2.   As a general rule:

            a.   Ocular motor cranial nerve palsy in young patient—greater likelihood of neoplasm; aggressive workup

            b.   Ocular motor cranial nerve palsy in older patient—greater likelihood of ischemic mononeuropathy; less aggressive workup

        3.   Note in series by Robertson and Kodsi (Table 4-1) that if cases due to trauma are excluded, a child with a VI nerve palsy has a 50-50 chance of harboring a neoplasm, usually a brainstem glioma

        4.   In pediatric patients, the syndrome of benign, postviral VI nerve palsy may occur:

            a.   Acute onset

            b.   Usually complete absence of abduction

            c.   Antecedent febrile viral illness

            d.   Absence of other cranial nerve dysfunction

            e.   No signs of increased intracranial pressure

            f.   Complete resolution within 3 months

            g.   May be recurrent

            h.   Careful follow-up mandatory

    B.   Initial evaluation

        1.   Blood pressure determination

        2.   Blood tests

            a.   Complete blood count (CBC)

            b.   Glucose tolerance test (GTT); hemoglobin A1C level

            c.   Sedimentation rate

            d.   VDRL and FTA-ABS (or TPHA)

            e.   Antinuclear antibody (ANA)

         3.   Radiographic studies

            a.   Patients under age 50 should undergo cranial magnetic resonance imaging (MRI)

            b.   In patients over age 50, the most likely cause is an ischemic mononeuropathy. If the VI nerve palsy has not resolved in 3 months, or if other cranial nerve involvement occurs, then comprehensive evaluation is recommended

                i.   Medical and neurologic examinations

                ii.   MRI

                iii.   Noninvasive cerebrovascular studies: magnetic resonance angiography (MRA), magnetic resonance venography (MRV), computed tomographic angiography (CTA)

                iv.   Lumbar puncture

                v.   Cerebral angiography

| Table 4-1 | | | | | | | |

ETIOLOGIES OF ACQUIRED VI NERVE PALSY

	Rucker (1958)	Schrader (1960) (isolated VI)	Rucker (1966)	Johnston (1968)	Robertson (1970) (children)	Rush (1981)	Kodsi (1992) (children)	Richards (1992)
Total # Patients	545	104	607	158	133	419	88	575
Etiologies (%)								
Neoplasm	21	7	33	13	39	15	21	20
Trauma	16	3	12	32	20	17	42	20
Aneurysm	6	0	3	1	3	3	0	3
Ischemic	11	36	8	16	0	18	0	10
Misc	16	30	24	30	29	18	22	23
Undetermined	30	24	20	8	9	29	15	23

VIII. Table 4-1 contains a summary of eight retrospective studies of patients with paresis of the VI nerve

  A. Eight to 30%, etiology undetermined, reflecting the vulnerability of the nerve to influences that are transient, benign, and unrecognizable

  B. Sixteen to 30% attributed to a miscellaneous group of causes that includes leukemia, migraine, pseudotumor cerebri, and multiple sclerosis. The miscellaneous group of etiologies reflects the poor localizing value of paresis of the VI nerve

IX. The six impostors of the VI nerve

  A. Thyroid eye disease

  B. Myasthenia gravis

  C. Duane's syndrome

  D. Spasm of the near reflex

  E. Medial wall orbital blowout fracture with restrictive myopathy

  F. Break in fusion of a congenital esophoria

BIBLIOGRAPHY

Chapters

Glaser JS, Siatkowski RM. Infranuclear disorders of eye movement. In: Glaser JS. *Neuro-Ophthalmology.* 3rd ed. Philadelphia, Pa: Lippincott William & Wilkins; 1999:405-460.

Leigh RJ, Zee DS. *The Neurology of Eye Movements.* 4th ed. New York, NY: Oxford University Press; 2006:385-474.

Sargent JC. Nuclear and and infranuclear ocular motility disorders. In: Miller NR, Newman NJ, eds. *Walsh and Hoyt's Clinical Neuro-Ophthalmology.* 6th ed. Vol 1. Philadelphia, Pa: Lippincott Williams & Wilkins; 2005:969-1040.

Articles

Cohen HA, Nussinovitch M, Askenazi A, et al. Benign abducens nerve palsy of childhood. *Pediatr Neurol.* 1993;9:394-395.

Duane A. Congenital deficiency of abduction associated with impairment of adduction, retraction movements, contraction of the palpebral fissure, and oblique movements of the eye. *Arch Ophthalmol.* 1905;34:133-159.

Gradenigo G. A special syndrome of endocranial otitic complications (paralysis of the motor oculi externus of otitic origin). *Ann Otol.* 1904;13:637.

Hotchkiss MG, Miller NR, Clark AW, et al. Bilateral Duane's retraction syndrome. A clinical pathologic case report. *Arch Ophthalmol.* 1980;98:870-874.

Jacobson DM. Progressive ophthalmoplegia with acute ischemic abducens palsies. *Am J Ophthalmol.* 1996;122:278-279.

Knox D, Clark D, Schuster F. Benign VI nerve palsies in children. *Pediatrics.* 1967;40:560-564.

Kodsi SR, Younge BR. Acquired oculomotor, trochlear, abducent cranial nerve palsies in pediatric patients. *Am J Ophthalmol.* 1992;114:568-574.

Lee MS, Galetta SL, Volpe NJ, Liu GT. Sixth nerve palsies in children. *Pediatr Neurol.* 1999;20:49-52.

Peters GB, Bakri SJ, Krohel GB. Cause and prognosis of nontraumatic sixth nerve palsies in young adults. *Ophthalmology.* 2002;109:1925-1928.

Richards BW, Jones FR, Young BR. Causes and prognosis in 4278 cases of paralysis of the oculomotor, trochlear, and abducens cranial nerves. *Am J Ophthalmol.* 1992;113:489-496.

Robertson DM, Hines JD, Rucker CW. Acquired sixth nerve paresis in children. *Arch Ophthalmol.* 1970;83:574-579.

Rucker CW. Paralysis of the third, fourth, and sixth cranial nerves. *Am J Ophthalmol.* 1958;46:787-794.

Rucker CW. The causes of paralysis of the third, fourth, and sixth cranial nerves. *Am J Ophthalmol.* 1966;61:1293-1298.

Rush JA, Younge BR. Paralysis of cranial nerves III, IV and VI. Cause and prognosis in 1,000 cases. *Arch Ophthalmol.* 1981;99:76-79.

Volpe NJ, Lessell S. Remitting sixth nerve palsy in skull base tumors. *Arch Ophthamol.* 1993;111:1391-1395.

Chapter 5

The Seven Syndromes of the III Nerve (Oculomotor)

Lanning B. Kline, MD

I. **Anatomical considerations**

    A.   Figure 5-1 represents a cross-section through the rostral midbrain at the level of the superior colliculi

    B.   Figure 5-2 is a copy of Figure 5-1 with superimposition of sites 1 through 6, representing six sites in which the III cranial nerve may be affected and present with distinct ocular manifestations, or in the company of different neurologic signs and symptoms, or as a result of specific disease processes. The seventh syndrome is the isolated III nerve palsy

    C.   Figure 5-3 illustrates the relationship of the III nerve (highlighted in black) to other cranial nerves

II. **The seven syndromes of the III nerve**

    A.   Nuclear III nerve paresis (see Figure 5-2, site 1)

        1.   Extremely rare

        2.   The arrangement of the III nerve subnuclei places strict prerequisites on the diagnosis of a nuclear III nerve palsy

            a.   Each superior rectus is innervated by the contralateral III nerve nucleus; therefore, a nuclear III nerve palsy on one side requires paresis of the contralateral superior rectus

            b.   Both levators are innervated by one subnuclear structure—the central caudal nucleus; therefore, a nuclear III nerve palsy requires bilateral ptosis

        3.   Some cases of skew deviation may actually represent instances of one or more III nerve subnuclei (subserving the vertical recti or the inferior oblique) being affected (see Chapter 2)

    B.   III nerve fascicle syndrome (see Figure 5-2, site 2)

        1.   Topical diagnosis depends upon the coexistence of other neurologic signs

        2.   Fascicles have already left the III nerve nucleus so that the ocular manifestations are present only on one side (no longer subject to the rules governing nuclear III nerve paresis)

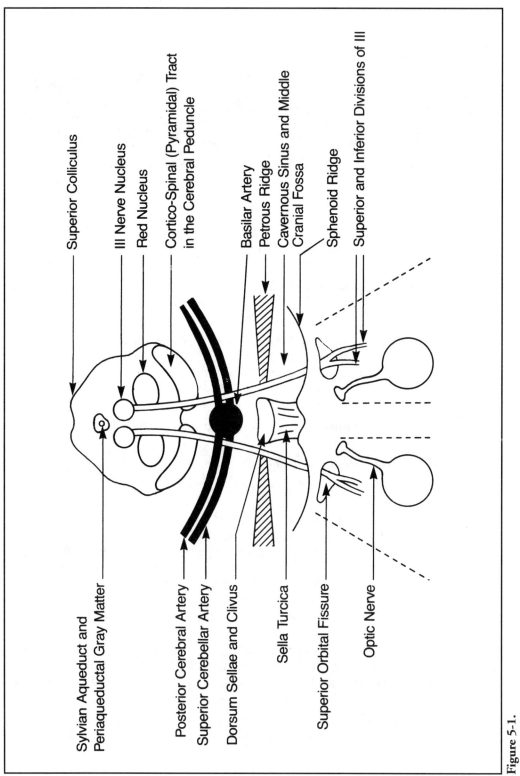

Figure 5-1.

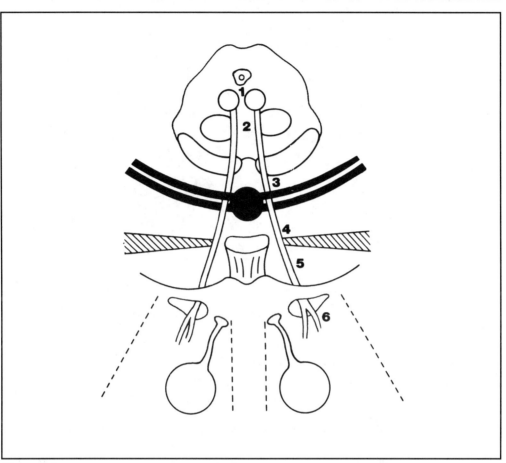

 Figure 5-2.

3.   Nothnagel's syndrome
  a.   Lesion in the area of the superior cerebellar peduncle
  b.   Ipsilateral III nerve paresis and cerebellar ataxia
4.   Benedikt's syndrome
  a.   Lesion in the region of the red nucleus
  b.   Ipsilateral III nerve paresis with contralateral hemitremor
5.   Weber's syndrome
  a.   Involvement of the III nerve in the neighborhood of the cerebral peduncle
  b.   Ipsilateral III nerve paresis with contralateral hemiparesis
6.   Claude's syndrome
  a.   Features of both Benedikt's and Nothnagel's syndromes
7.   Fascicular lesions are virtually always ischemic, infiltrative (tumor), or rarely inflammatory
C.   Uncal herniation syndrome (see Figure 5-2, site 3)
  1.   In its course toward the cavernous sinus, the III nerve rests on the edge of the tentorium cerebelli

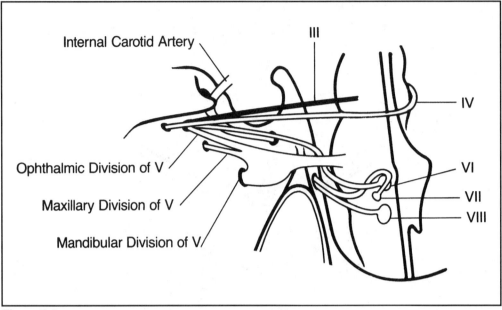

Internal Carotid Artery

III

IV

Ophthalmic Division of V

VI

VII

VIII

Maxillary Division of V

Mandibular Division of V

Figure 5-3.

2. The portion of the brain overlying the III nerve, at the tentorial edge, is the uncal portion of the undersurface of the temporal lobe

3. A supratentorial space-occupying mass, located anywhere in or above this cerebral hemisphere, may cause a downward displacement and herniation of the uncus across the tentorial edge, thereby compressing the III nerve (Figure 5-4)

4. A dilated and fixed pupil (Hutchinson pupil) may be the first indication that altered consciousness is due to a space-occupying intracranial lesion

D. Posterior communicating artery aneurysm (see Figure 5-2, site 4)

1. In its course toward the cavernous sinus, the III nerve travels alongside (lateral to) the posterior communicating artery

2. The most common cause of nontraumatic isolated III nerve paresis with pupillary involvement is an aneurysm at the junction of the posterior communicating artery and the internal carotid artery (Figure 5-5)

3. Hemorrhage suddenly enlarges the aneurysmal sac to which the III nerve is adherent or there is actual hemorrhage into the substance of the nerve

4. On occasion, the pupil is spared early in the course of aneurysmal compression of the III nerve. The patient must be followed carefully during the initial 5 to 7 days to be certain of the status of the pupil

E. Cavernous sinus syndrome (see Figure 5-2, site 5)

1. III nerve paresis is usually seen in association with other cranial nerve involvement: IV, V, VI, and oculosympathetic paralysis

2. III nerve paresis due to cavernous sinus lesion tends to be partial (ie, all muscles innervated by the III nerve are not equally involved)

3. Pupillary fibers are frequently "spared," such that the pupil may be normal or minimally involved

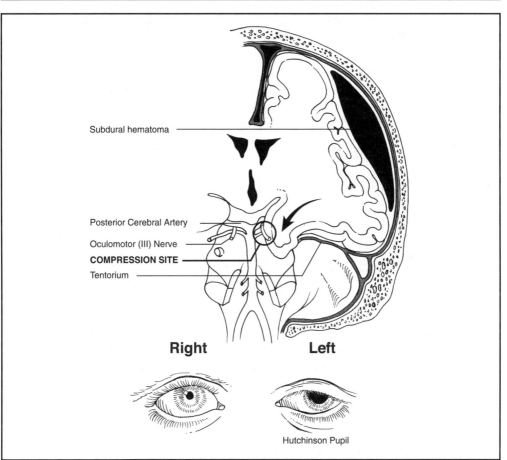

Figure 5-4. Transtentorial herniation of the uncus of the temporal lobe with III nerve compression.

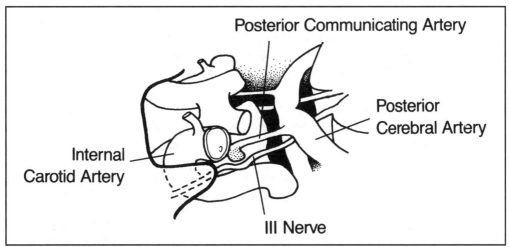

Figure 5-5. Compression of the left III nerve due to aneurysm at the junction of the posterior communicating and internal carotid arteries.

4. Cavernous sinus lesions may lead to primary aberrant regeneration of the III nerve (see below)

5. See Chapter 7

F. Orbital syndrome (see Figure 5-2, site 6)

1. See the orbital syndrome of the VI nerve (see Chapter 4)

2. Just before entering the superior orbital fissure, the III nerve splits into two divisions

3. The superior division innervates the:

   a. Superior rectus

   b. Levator palpebrae

4. The inferior division innervates the:

   a. Inferior rectus

   b. Medial rectus

   c. Inferior oblique

   d. Pupil (iris sphincter muscle)

   e. Accommodation (ciliary muscle)

5. Orbital involvement of the III nerve may result in selective paresis of structures innervated by only one of the divisions

G. Pupil-sparing isolated III nerve paresis (the seventh syndrome of the III nerve)

1. The pupillomotor fibers of the III nerve travel in the outer layers of the nerve and are therefore closer to the nutrient blood supply enveloping the nerve (Figure 5-6)

2. This may explain why the pupillomotor fibers are spared in 80% of ischemic III nerve pareses but are affected in 95% of cases of compressive (trauma, tumor, aneurysm) III nerve paresis

3. Patients with pupil-sparing isolated III nerve palsies are evaluated and managed in a similar manner to patients with isolated IV and VI nerve pareses

   a. Ischemia lab workup

      i. Blood pressure determination

      ii. Complete blood count (CBC)

      iii. Sedimentation rate

      iv. Glucose tolerance test (GTT); hemoglobin A1C

      v. VDRL and FTA-ABS (or TPHA)

      vi. ANA (antinuclear antibody)

   b. Follow the patient for 3 months if:

      i. The III nerve paresis is truly isolated

      ii. The patient is over 50 years of age

      iii. The patient has a history of diabetes or hypertension

   c. Most patients with ischemic III nerve paresis demonstrate improvement of the motility measurements within 1 month and complete recovery by 3 months

   d. Recommend cranial magnetic resonance imaging (MRI), magnetic resonance angiography (MRA), computed tomographic angiography (CTA), possibly lumbar puncture, and four-vessel cerebral angiography if:

      i. The pupil becomes dilated in the initial 5 to 7 days after onset

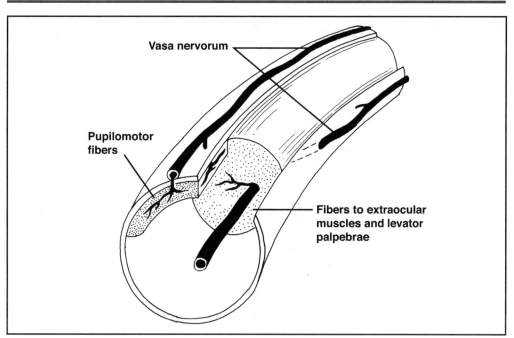

Figure 5-6. Blood supply to portions of III nerve supplying the pupil and extraocular muscles.

        ii.   No significant improvement in 3 months

        iii.   The patient develops signs of aberrant regeneration of the III nerve

        iv.   Other neurologic findings develop

   e.   **Caution:** ocular myasthenia can mimic a pupil-sparing III nerve palsy; remember the Tensilon test!

H.   Diagnostic guidelines for patient with isolated III nerve palsy

   1.   While the size and reactivity of the pupil are major determinants in patient evaluation, other important considerations include:

      a.   Age of patient (see Chapter 5, III, C)

      b.   Degree of somatic (motility, lid) involvement

      c.   Some pupillary involvement (<2 mm anisocoria) is found in up to one third of patients with ischemic (eg, diabetic) III nerve palsies

      d.   Pupillary involvement may develop during the initial 5 to 7 days of a compressive III nerve palsy

      e.   Periorbital pain does not reliably distinguish between compressive vs vasculopathic etiology

   2.   Guidelines:

      a.   All children less than 10 years (no matter the pupillary findings) should undergo MRI, MRA, and CTA. If normal, proceed with cerebral angiography

      b.   All patients older than 10 years with pupil-involving III nerve palsy should undergo MRI, MRA, and CTA. Depending on results, may need cerebral angiography

	Table 5-1						

ETIOLOGIES OF ACQUIRED III NERVE PALSY

	Rucker (1958)	Goldstein (1960) (isolated III)	Green (1964)	Rucker (1966)	Rush (1981)	Kodsi (1992) (children)	Richards (1992)	Schumacher-Feero (1999) (children)
Total # Patients	335	61	130	274	290	35	244	49
Etiologies (%)								
Neoplasm	11	10	4	18	12	14	10	12
Trauma	15	8	11	13	16	40	14	31
Aneurysm	19	18	30	18	14	0	12	8
Ischemic*	19	47	19	17	21	0	23	0
Misc	8	6	13	12	14	29	18	47
Undetermined	28	11	23	20	23	17	23	2

*Including diabetes mellitus.

    c.   All patients 10 to 50 years with pupil-sparing III nerve palsy should undergo MRI and MRA. If normal:

        i.   Medical evaluation—diabetes mellitus, hypertension

        ii.   Observe for pupillary involvement

        iii.   Follow for development of other neurologic abnormalities

    d.   All patients 50 years and older with pupil-sparing III nerve palsy with total somatic involvement:

        i.   Observation

        ii.   Medical work-up—diabetes mellitus, hypertension, giant cell arteritis

    e.   All patients 50 years and older with partial pupillary involvement (anisocoria >2 mm but pupil not fixed and dilated) should undergo MRI, MRA, and CTA. If results are normal, strongly consider cerebral angiography

III.   Incidence of various causes of III nerve palsies

    A.   Table 5-1 summarizes eight major published series of patients with paresis of the oculomotor nerve

    B.   Although neoplasm, aneurysm, and ischemia are the most common etiologies, approximately 10% to 25% of cases of III nerve palsies have an undetermined cause

    C.   Approximately one half of III nerve palsies in children are congenital and a high percentage have signs of aberrant regeneration. However, approximately 10% to 20% are due to aneurysm or neoplasm; therefore, all children should undergo MR scanning

IV.   Aberrant regeneration (misdirection) of the III nerve

A. Regeneration of the disrupted III nerve fibers may result in fibers of one structure being hooked up ("axon sprouting") to fibers that terminate in another structure

B. Clinical phenomena may be classified as:
    1. Lid-gaze dyskinesis
        a. Some of the inferior rectus fibers may end up innervating the levator so that the lid retracts when the patient looks down: pseudo-von Graefe's sign
        b. Some of the medial rectus fibers may end up supplying some of the innervation to the levator so that the lid retracts when the patient adducts his or her eye: inverse Duane's syndrome
    2. Pupil-gaze dyskinesis
        a. Some of the medial rectus fibers may end up innervating the pupillary sphincter muscle so that there is more pupil constriction during convergence than as a response to light: pseudo-Argyll Robertson pupil
        b. Some of the fibers destined to innervate the inferior rectus may end up innervating the pupillary sphincter so that on attempted downgaze, the pupil constricts

C. Two forms of aberrant regeneration are:
    1. Primary aberrant regeneration
        a. No preceding acute III nerve palsy
        b. Insidious development of III nerve palsy with accompanying signs of misdirection
        c. Sign of an intracavernous lesion: meningioma, aneurysm, neurinoma
    2. Secondary aberrant regeneration
        a. Observe weeks to months during recovery from a III nerve palsy
        b. Seen after trauma and tumor compression of the III nerve, but never after ischemic III nerve paresis. If you are following a patient with a presumed diagnosis of ischemic III nerve palsy and he or she develops signs of aberrant regeneration, then MR scanning and cerebral angiography are indicated

V. Rare causes of III nerve palsy

A. Minor head trauma
    1. In general, head trauma causing III nerve palsy is severe enough to cause loss of consciousness and often other neurologic deficits
    2. Rarely, a patient may harbor a basal intracranial tumor and, with only minor head trauma, develop a III nerve palsy
    3. Minimal head injury resulting in a III nerve palsy is an indication for cranial MRI

B. Ophthalmoplegic migraine (see Chapter 15, V, I)
    1. Onset almost always in childhood
    2. Usually a family history of migraine
    3. III nerve palsy may occur at any time in relation to headache but usually appears as the headache phase abates
    4. As a rule, III nerve palsy clears completely within 1 month, but occasionally permanent oculomotor paresis occurs

5. MRI may demonstrate thickening and enhancement of cisternal (site 3) portion of III nerve
6. Pathophysiology uncertain: ischemia, inflammation, demyelination
7. Disorder may be mimicked by mass lesion (schwannoma, angioma) of III nerve

C. Cyclic oculomotor palsy
1. Disorder usually present at birth or in early childhood
2. Occurs in the setting of a total III nerve palsy
3. Spastic movements of the muscles innervated by the III nerve results in lid elevation, adduction, miosis, and increased accommodation
4. These movements occur at regular intervals, lasting 10 to 30 seconds
5. Etiology unknown

BIBLIOGRAPHY

Chapters

Glaser JS, Siatkowski RM. Infranuclear disorders of eye movements. In: Glaser JS. *Neuro-Ophthalmology*. 3rd ed. Philadelphia, Pa: Lippincott Williams & Wilkins; 1999:405-460.

Leigh RJ, Zee DS. *The Neurology of Eye Movements*. 4th ed. New York, NY: Oxford University Press; 2006:385-474.

Sargent JC. Nuclear and infranuclear ocular motility disorders. In: Miller NR, Newman NJ, eds. *Walsh and Hoyt's Clinical Neuro-Ophthalmology*. 6th ed. Vol 1. Philadelphia, Pa: Lippincott Williams & Wilkins; 2005:969-1040.

Articles

Angel BG, Antonio MS, Jesus PE, et al. Venous angioma associated with atypical ophthalmoplegic migraine. *Headache*. 2004;44:440-442.

Asbury AK, Aldredge H, Hirshberg R, et al. Oculomotor palsy in diabetes mellitus: a clinicopathological study. *Brain*. 1970;93:555-566.

Cox TA, Wurster IB, Godfrey WA. Primary aberrant oculomotor regeneration due to intracranial aneurysm. *Arch Neurol*. 1979;36:570-571.

Eyster EF, Hoyt WF, Wilson CB. Oculomotor palsy from minor head trauma. An initial sign of basal intracranial tumor. *JAMA*. 1972;220:1083-1086.

Friedman AP, Harter DH, Merritt HH. Ophthalmoplegic migraine. *Arch Neurol*. 1962;7:320-327.

Goldstein JE, Cogan DG. Diabetic ophthalmoplegia with special reference to the pupil. *Arch Ophthalmol*. 1960;64:592-600.

Green WR, Hackett ER, Schlezinger NS. Neuro-ophthalmic evaluation of oculomotor nerve paralysis. *Arch Ophthalmol*. 1964;72:154-167.

Harley RD. Paralytic strabismus in children: etiologic incidence and management of the third, fourth, and sixth nerve palsies. *Ophthalmology*. 1980;87:24-43.

Hopf HC, Gutman L. Diabetic third nerve palsy: evidence for a mesencephalic lesion. *Neurology*. 1990;40:1041-1045.

Jacobson DM. Pupil involvement in patients with diabetes-associated oculomotor nerve palsy. *Arch Ophthalmol*. 1998;116:723-727.

Jacobson DM, Broste SK. Early progression of ophthalmoplegia in patients with ischemic oculomotor nerve palsies. *Arch Ophthalmol.* 1995;113:1525-1537.

Kissel JT, Burde RM, Klingele TG, et al. Pupil-sparing oculomotor palsies with internal carotid-posterior communicating artery aneurysms. *Ann Neurol.* 1983;13:149-154.

Kodsi SR, Younge BR. Acquired oculomotor, trochlear and abducent cranial nerve palsies in pediatric patients. *Am J Ophthalmol.* 1992;114:568-574.

Lepore FE, Glaser JS. Misdirection revisited: a critical appraisal of acquired oculomotor nerve synkinesis. *Arch Ophthalmol.* 1980;98:2206-2209.

Loewenfeld IE, Thompson HS. Oculomotor paresis with cyclical spasms. A critical review of the literature and a new case. *Arch Ophthalmol.* 1975;20:81-124.

Murakami T, Funatsuka M, Kamine M, et al. Oculomotor nerve schwannoma mimicking ophthalmoplegic migraine. *Neuropediatrics.* 2005;36:395-398.

Richards BW, Jones FR, Younge BR. Causes and prognosis in 4278 cases of paralysis of the oculomotor, trochlear and abducens cranial nerves. *Am J Ophthalmol.* 1992;113:489-496.

Rucker CW. Paralysis of the third, fourth, and sixth cranial nerves. *Am J Ophthalmol.* 1958;46:787-794.

Rucker CW. The causes of paralysis of the third, fourth, and sixth cranial nerves. *Am J Ophthalmol.* 1966;61:1293-1298.

Rush JA, Younge BR. Paralysis of cranial nerves III, IV, and VI. Cause and prognosis in 1,000 cases. *Arch Ophthalmol.* 1981;99:76-79.

Schatz NJ, Savino PJ, Corbett JJ. Primary aberrant oculomotor regeneration. A sign of intracavernous meningioma. *Arch Neurol.* 1977;34:29-32.

Schumacher-Feero LA, Yoo KW, Solari FM, et al. Third cranial nerve palsy in children. *Am J Ophthalmol.* 1999;128:216-221.

Trobe JD. Managing oculomotor nerve palsy. *Arch Ophthalmol.* 1998;116:798.

Weber RB, Daroff RB, Mackey EM. Pathology of oculomotor nerve palsy in diabetics. *Neurology.* 1970;20:835-838.

Chapter 6

The Five Syndromes of the IV Nerve (Trochlear)

Lanning B. Kline, MD

I.   **Anatomical considerations**

   A.   Figure 6-1 is a diagram of a cross-section of the lower midbrain at the level of the inferior colliculi

   B.   The IV nerve is:
   1.   The only cranial nerve that exits at the dorsal aspect of the brainstem (Figure 6-2)
   2.   The cranial nerve with the longest intracranial course (75 mm)

   C.   The IV nerve fascicles cross in the anterior medullary velum (roof of the Sylvian aqueduct) prior to exiting dorsally and coursing anteriorly around the midbrain to travel forward between the superior cerebellar and posterior cerebral arteries (just as, but laterally separated from, the III cranial nerve)

   D.   Therefore, the left IV nerve fascicle becomes the right IV nerve and innervates the right superior oblique muscle; and the right IV nerve fascicle becomes the left IV nerve and innervates the left superior oblique muscle

II.   **Clinical syndromes of the IV nerve (Figure 6-3): nuclear-fascicular syndrome, subarachnoid space syndrome, cavernous sinus syndrome, orbital syndrome, isolated IV nerve palsy (congenital or acquired)**

   A.   Nuclear-fascicular syndrome (see Figure 6-3, site 1)
   1.   Distinguishing nuclear from fascicular lesions is virtually impossible due to the short course of the fascicles within the midbrain, thus the lack of associated neurologic signs
   2.   Frequent etiologies include hemorrhage, infarction, demyelination, trauma (including neurosurgical)
   3.   Fascicular lesion may be seen with contralateral Horner's syndrome, since the sympathetic pathways descend through the dorsolateral tegmentum of the midbrain adjacent to the trochlear fascicles

   B.   Subarachnoid space syndrome (see Figure 6-3, site 2)
   1.   IV nerve particularly susceptible to injury as it emerges from the dorsal surface of brainstem

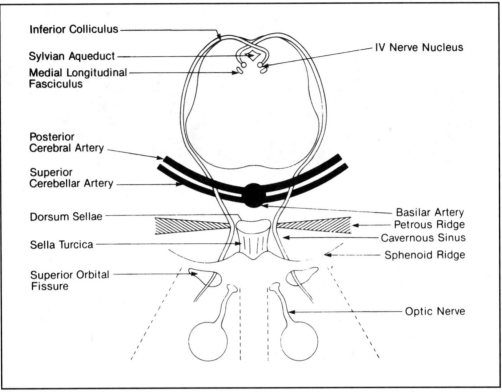

Figure 6-1.

2.   When bilateral IV nerve palsies occur, the site of injury is likely in the anterior medullary velum. Contrecoup forces transmitted to the brainstem by the free tentorial edge may injure the nerves at this site

3.   Less frequent causes include tumor (eg, pinealoma, tentorial meningioma), meningitis, neurosurgical trauma

C.   Cavernous sinus syndrome (see Figure 6-3, site 3)

1.   Seen in association with other cranial nerve palsies: III, V, VI oculosympathetic paralysis

2.   Checking IV nerve function in the setting of a III nerve paresis

a.   Since the involved eye cannot be adducted well, the vertical actions of the superior oblique muscle cannot be tested

b.   Therefore, the eye is moved into abduction and then the patient is instructed to look down; the ability of the eye to intort is examined as a measure of IV nerve function

c.   If a limbal or conjunctival landmark (eg, pterygium or blood vessel) is noted to intort, then the IV nerve is presumed intact

3.   See Chapter 7

D.   Orbital syndrome (see Figure 6-3, site 4)

1.   Usually seen in association with III, IV, and VI cranial nerve palsies: orbital signs including proptosis, chemosis, conjunctival injection

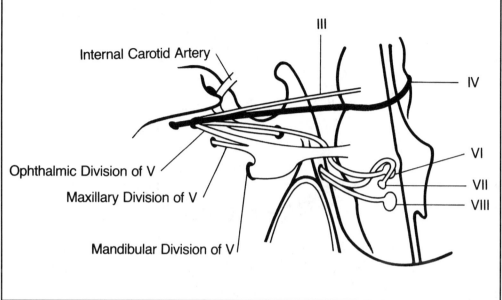

Figure 6-2. Diagram of the IV nerve (highlighted in black) and its relationship to cranial nerves III through VIII.

       2.   Major etiologies include trauma, inflammation, tumor

  E.   Isolated IV nerve palsy (the fifth syndrome of the IV nerve)

       1.   Congenital

          a.   See Chapter 6, VI for incidence of this condition

          b.   Most often seen in pediatric population and late in life (fifth to seventh decades) as patient's IV nerve palsy may decompensate

          c.   Diagnostic keys

              i.   Large vertical fusion amplitude (10 to 15 prism diopters)

             ii.   FAT (family album tomography) scan: look at old photographs to detect long-standing head tilt, indicative of congenital etiology

       2.   Acquired

          a.   Acute onset of vertical diplopia, usually with torsional component

          b.   Characteristic head position

              i.   Tilt to opposite shoulder

             ii.   Head turned downward with chin depressed, eyes up

             iii.   Face turned to opposite side

          c.   Must perform Parks-Bielschowsky three-step test (see below) to confirm diagnosis

          d.   Initial evaluation

              i.   Blood pressure determination

             ii.   Glucose tolerance test (GTT); hemoglobin A1C

             iii.   Sedimentation rate

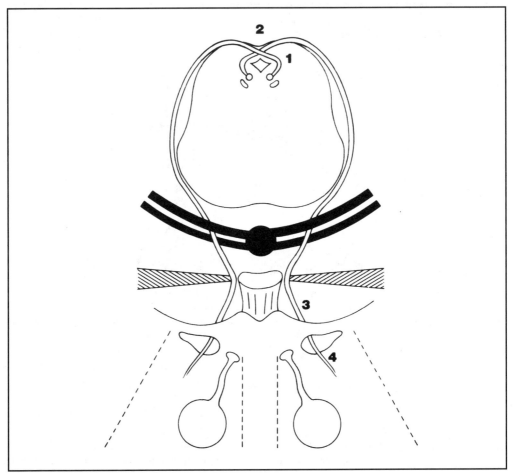

Figure 6-3. Clinical syndromes of the IV nerve.

      e.   As with other isolated ocular motor neuropathies, if the IV nerve palsy has not improved or resolved within 3 months, or if other neurologic signs develop, further workup is indicated

          i.   Medical and neurologic examinations

          ii.   Magnetic resonance imaging (MRI)

          iii.   Cerebrovascular studies: magnetic resonance angiography (MRA), magnetic resonance venography (MRV), computed tomographic angiography (CTA), cerebral angiography

          iv.   Lumbar puncture

III. Diagnosis of recently acquired IV nerve palsy

    A.   If a patient has vertical misalignment (hypertropia [HT]) due to recently acquired weakness of a single vertically acting muscle, then determine the weak muscle by performing the Parks-Bielschowsky three-step test (Figure 6-4)

        1.   The medial and lateral rectus muscles do not have vertical action

        2.   Therefore, HT of paretic etiology is caused by weakness of one or more of the following eight vertically acting muscles:

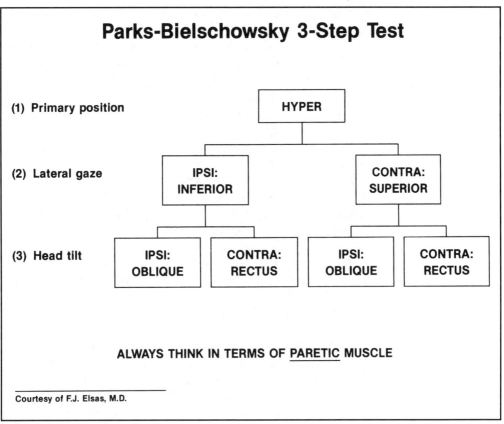

Figure 6-4.

    a.   Right inferior oblique (RIO); left inferior oblique (LIO)

    b.   Right superior oblique (RSO); left superior oblique (LSO)

    c.   Right inferior rectus (RIR); left inferior rectus (LIR)

    d.   Right superior rectus (RSR); left superior rectus (LSR)

3.   If the HT is due to weakness of only one of these eight muscles, the paretic muscle is identified by answering the three questions asked in the Parks-Bielschowsky three-step test

4.   Each step cuts the possible number of muscles in half

    a.   After the first step, there are four possible muscles remaining

    b.   After the second step, there are two remaining

    c.   After the third step, only the one guilty muscle remains

5.   Parks-Bielschowsky first step: which is the higher eye?

    a.   If the patient has a RHT, then the weak muscle is either a depressor of the right eye (RIR, RSO) or an elevator of the left eye (LSR, LIO)

    b.   If the patient has a LHT, then the weak muscle is either an elevator of the right eye (RSR, RIO) or a depressor of the left eye (LIR, LSO)

    c.   Therefore, by determining if the patient has a RHT or a LHT, you have narrowed down the number of suspected muscles from eight to four

6.   Parks-Bielschowsky second step: HT worse on gaze right or left?

   a.   The vertical rectus muscles (superior and inferior recti) have their greatest vertical action (and least torsional action) when the eye is abducted

   b.   Therefore, LHT due to paresis of LIR will be worse on gaze left (since OS is abducted on gaze left); LHT due to paresis of RSR will be worse on gaze right (since OD is abducted on right gaze)

   c.   The oblique muscles (superior and inferior obliques) have their greatest vertical action (and least torsional action) when the eye is adducted

   d.   Therefore, LHT due to paresis of LSO will be worse on gaze right; LHT due to paresis of RIO will be worse on gaze left

   e.   LHT worse on gaze right is due to weakness of either LSO or RSR

   f.   LHT worse on gaze left is due to weakness of either LIR or RIO

   g.   Thus, in the case of LHT, by answering the question: "Is LHT worse on gaze right or left?" you have narrowed the possible muscles from four (LSO, RSR, LIR, RIO) to two (either LSO-RSR or LIR-RIO)

   h.   Similarly, the possible causes of RHT are narrowed down from four (RIR, LIO, LSR, RSO) to two (RIR-LIO if RHT worse on gaze right; RSO-LSR if RHT worse on gaze left). Note: in each case

      i.   RHT worse on gaze right (RIR or LIO)

      ii.   RHT worse on gaze left (RSO or LSR)

      iii.   LHT worse on gaze right (LSO or RSR)

      iv.   LHT worse on gaze left (LIR or RIO)

      You are left with either two superior or two inferior muscles; and one will be a rectus and one an oblique, and one will be of the right eye and one of the left. If this is not the case (eg, if you have narrowed it down after the second step to "RIR vs LSR" or "LSO vs LIO"), then you have made a mistake and need to retrace your steps

7.   Parks-Bielschowsky third step: is the HT worse on head-tilt right (head tilted so that the right ear is near the right shoulder) or head-tilt left (head tilted so that the left ear is near the left shoulder)?

   a.   The superior muscles (SR and SO) intort the eyes; the inferior muscles (IR and IO) extort the eye

   b.   When the head is tilted downward to the right shoulder, the eyes undergo corrective torsion (ie, OD intorted and OS extorted)

   c.   Therefore, when the head is tilted to the right, OD will be intorted by contraction of RSR and RSO; these two muscles work together in affecting the intorsion and neutralize each other's vertical action (RSR is an elevator and RSO a depressor)

   d.   If one of these muscles is the paretic muscle responsible for the HT, then the vertical action will not be neutralized and the HT will be worse on tilting the head to the right shoulder

   e.   Therefore, the mnemonic for the third step is:

      i.   If you are left with two superior muscles, then the paretic muscle is the one on the same side as the shoulder toward which the head-tilt makes the HT worse (eg, if it is narrowed down to "RSO vs LSR," then the paretic muscle is "RSO if RHT worse on tilt to right" and "LSR if RHT is worse to tilt left")

        ii.   If you are left with two inferior muscles, then the paretic muscle is the one on the side opposite the shoulder toward which the head-tilt makes the HT worse (eg, if it is narrowed down to "RIO vs LIR," then the paretic muscle is "RIO if LHT worse on tilt left" and "LIR if LHT worse on tilt right")

  B.   Bajandas described Bielschowsky's "missing step": is the HT worse on gaze up or gaze down?

      1.   This step confirms step three

      2.   Note again that after step two we are down to either two superior or two inferior muscles

          a.   RSR vs LSO

          b.   RSO vs LSR

          c.   RIR vs LIO

          d.   RIO vs LIR

      3.   Note also that in each case, one muscle is an elevator and the other a depressor

      4.   Therefore, we can confirm the paretic muscle identified by step three by noting if the HT is worse on gaze up (RSR, LSR, LIO, RIO) or gaze down (LSO, RSO, RIR, LIR)

IV.   Measuring the torsional component of IV nerve palsy

  A.   Double Maddox rod test to quantitate torsional component of diplopia

  B.   The patient will report intorsion of image seen by eye with IV nerve palsy. Actually, this indicates extorsion of the patient's eye caused by overaction of the antagonist inferior oblique muscle (Figure 6-5)

  C.   Greater than 10 degrees of torsion is suggestive of bilateral IV nerve palsies

V.   Bilateral IV nerve palsies

  A.   Usually due to severe head trauma with contusion of the anterior medullary velum where the IV nerve fascicles cross

  B.   Parks-Bielschowsky three-step test

      1.   Either eye may be hypertropic in primary position or patient may be orthophoric

      2.   RHT on gaze left; LHT on gaze right

      3.   RHT on head-tilt right; LHT on head-tilt left

  C.   With double Maddox rods, measure greater than 10 degrees of torsion

VI. Incidence of various causes of IV nerve palsy

  A.   Table 6-1 summarizes eight large series of patients with acquired paresis of the IV nerve

  B.   Summary of cases of acquired, isolated IV paresis (10-20-30-40 rule)

      1.   10%: neoplasm-aneurysm

      2.   20%: ischemic

      3.   30%: undetermined or miscellaneous

      4.   40%: trauma

  C.   In addition to acquired causes, a large proportion of IV nerve palsies are classified as congenital. In various series of patients, the frequency of congenital IV nerve palsies ranges from 29% (Younge et al, 1977) to 67% (Harley, 1980)

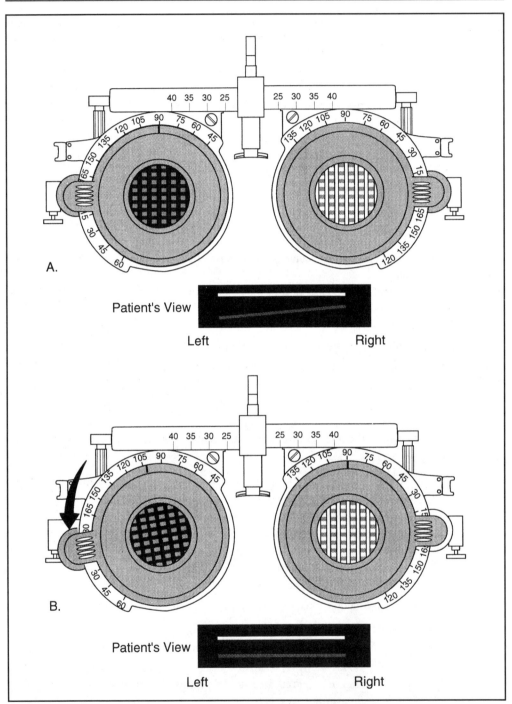

Figure 6-5. Double Maddox rod test for cyclodeviation in a patient with a right IV nerve palsy. A red and white Maddox rod is inserted into a trial frame, with the red lens before the eye with a suspected cyclodeviation. Special care must be taken to align the direction of the glass rods with the 90-degree mark of the trial frame. The trial frame must be adjusted carefully to a more exact horizontal position. (Modified from Van Noorden GK. *Atlas of Strabismus.* 4th ed. St Louis, Mo: CV Mosby; 1983:52-53.)

	Table 6-1							

ETIOLOGIES OF ACQUIRED IV NERVE PALSY

	Rucker (1958)	Rucker (1966)	Khawam (1967)	Burger (1970)	Younge (1977)	Rush (1981)	Kodsi (1992) (children)	Richards (1992)
Total # Patients	67	84	40	33	36	172	19	248
Etiologies (%)								
Neoplasm	4	8	2.5	21	0	4	5	4
Trauma	36	27	67.5	39	44	32	37	26
Aneurysm	0	0	0	3	0	2	0	1
Ischemic	36	15	2.5	18	33	18	0	14
Misc	10	15	7.5	9	8	4	37	20
Undetermined	13	33	20	6	15	36	21	35

    D.   The frequency of congenital IV nerve paresis cannot be overemphasized. Many adults presenting in the fifth and sixth decades of life may have decompensated, congenital IV nerve palsies

VII. Differential diagnosis of vertical diplopia

    A.   Ocular myasthenia

    B.   Thyroid eye disease

    C.   Orbital disease (tumor, trauma, inflammation, blowout fracture of the floor)

    D.   III nerve paresis

    E.   Brown's syndrome

    F.   Skew deviation

VIII. Other syndromes of the superior oblique muscle

    A.   Brown's (sheath) syndrome

        1.   Limitation of elevation of the eye in adduction because movements of the superior oblique tendon in the trochlea are restricted; elevation in abduction normal or near normal

        2.   Affected eyes usually hypotropic, and the patient often develops abnormal head position (chin up) and face turn (away from Brown's eye)

        3.   Forced ductions must be positive to establish diagnosis

        4.   Congenital etiology: superior oblique tendon is short and tethered

        5.   Acquired etiologies:

            a.   Tenosynovitis may prevent tendon from passing through the trochlear pulley

            b.   Orbital trauma to trochlear region

            c.   Superonasal orbital mass

    B.   Superior oblique myokymia

        1.   Unexplained condition causing vertical diplopia or monocular blurred vision with tremulous sensations of the affected eye

2. Paroxysmal, rapid, vertical, and torsional movements of one eye that are usually small, necessitating slit-lamp examination or ophthalmoscopy

3. Precipitated by asking the patient to first look in the direction of action of the superior oblique muscle and then return to the primary position

4. Usually benign; occasionally seen with multiple sclerosis or posterior fossa tumor

5. Treatment:

   a. Carbamazepine (Tegretol [Novartis Pharmaceuticals Corp, East Hanover, NJ]); propranolol (Inderal [Wyeth, Madison, NJ]); gabapentin (Neurontin [Pfizer, New York, NY])

   b. Superior oblique surgery

BIBLIOGRAPHY

Chapters

Glaser JS, Siatkowski RM. Infranuclear disorders of eye movements. In: Glaser JS. *Neuro-Ophthalmology*. 3rd ed. Philadelphia, Pa: Lippincott Williams & Wilkins; 1999:405-460.

Leigh RJ, Zee DS. *The Neurology of Eye Movements*. 4th ed. New York, NY: Oxford University Press; 2006:385-474.

Sargent JC. Nuclear and infranuclear ocular motility disorders. In: Miller NR, Newman NJ, eds. *Walsh and Hoyt's Clinical Neuro-Ophthalmology*. 6th ed. Vol 1. Philadelphia, Pa: Lippincott Williams & Wilkins; 2005:969-1040.

Articles

Brown HW. True and simulated superior oblique tendon sheath syndromes. *Doc Ophthalmol*. 1973;34:123-136.

Coppeto IR. Superior oblique paresis and contralateral Horner's syndrome. *Ann Ophthalmol*. 1983;681-683.

Harley RD. Paralytic strabismus in children: etiologic incidence and management of the third, fourth, and sixth nerve palsies. *Ophthalmology*. 1980;86:24-43.

Hoyt WF, Keane JR. Superior oblique myokymia: report and discussion on five cases of benign intermittent uniocular microtremor. *Arch Ophthalmol*. 1970;84:461-467.

Jacobson DM, Warner JJ, Choucair AK, Ptacek LJ. Trochlear nerve palsy following minor head trauma. A sign of structural disorder. *Journal of Clinical Neuro-Ophthalmology*. 1988;8:263-268.

Kodsi SR, Younge BR. Acquired oculomotor trochlear and abducent cranial nerve palsies in pediatric patients. *Am J Ophthalmol*. 1992;114:568-574.

Morrow MJ, Sharpe JA, Ranalli PJ. Superior oblique myokymia associated with a posterior fossa tumor: oculographic correlation with an idiopathic case. *Neurology*. 1990;40:367-370.

Moster ML, Bosley TM, Slavin ML, Rubin SE. Thyroid ophthalmopathy presenting as superior oblique palsies. *Journal of Clinical Neuro-Ophthalmology*. 1992;12:94-97.

Parks MM. Isolated cyclovertical muscle palsy. *Arch Ophthalmol*. 1958;60:1027-1035.

Richards BW, Jones FR, Younge BR. Cause and prognoses of 4278 cases of paralysis of oculomotor, trochlear and abducens cranial nerves. *Am J Ophthalmol*. 1992;183:489-496.

Rucker CW. Paralysis of the third, fourth, and sixth cranial nerves. *Am J Ophthalmol*. 1958;46:787-794.

Rucker CW. The causes of paralysis of the third, fourth, and sixth cranial nerves. *Am J Ophthalmol.* 1966;61:1293-1298.

Rush JA, Younge BR. Paralysis of cranial nerves III, IV, and VI. Cause and prognosis in 1,000 cases. *Arch Ophthalmol.* 1981;99:76-79.

Tomsak RL, Kosmorsky GS, Leigh RJ. Gabapentin attenuates superior oblique myokymia. *Am J Ophthalmol.* 2002;133:721-723.

Younge BR, Sutula F. Analysis of trochlear nerve palsies. *Mayo Clin Proc.* 1977;52:11-18.

Yousry I, Dieterich M, Naidich TP, et al. Superior oblique myokymia: magnetic resonance imagery support for the neurovascular compression hypothesis. *Ann Neurol.* 2002;51:361-368.

Chapter 7

Cavernous Sinus Syndrome

Lanning B. Kline, MD

I. **General considerations**

   A. The ocular motor cranial nerves lie in proximity within the cavernous sinus and superior orbital fissure

   B. Since the cavernous sinus contains structures that continue through the superior orbital fissure, it is often impossible to state whether a lesion is in the sinus or in the fissure. More general designation is parasellar syndrome

   C. Typically, patients present with periorbital or hemicranial pain, combined with ipsilateral ocular motor cranial nerve palsies, oculosympathetic paralysis, and sensory loss in the distribution of the ophthalmic (V^1) and occasionally maxillary (V^2) division of the trigeminal nerve. Clinically, various combinations of these cranial nerve palsies occur

   D. The "orbital apex syndrome" should be reserved for multiple ocular motor cranial nerve palsies plus optic nerve dysfunction

II. **Anatomy (Figures 7-1 and 7-2)**

   A. Traditionally, the cavernous sinus was thought to be an unbroken, trabeculated structure, but recent studies demonstrate that it is a plexus of various-sized veins that divide and coalesce

   B. Major constituents:
      1. III nerve
      2. IV nerve
      3. VI nerve
      4. Ophthalmic nerve (V^1)
      5. Sympathetic carotid plexus
      6. Intracavernous carotid artery

   C. The III, IV, V^1 nerves all lie in a lateral wall of the cavernous sinus. The VI nerve lies freely within the sinus, just lateral to the intracavernous carotid

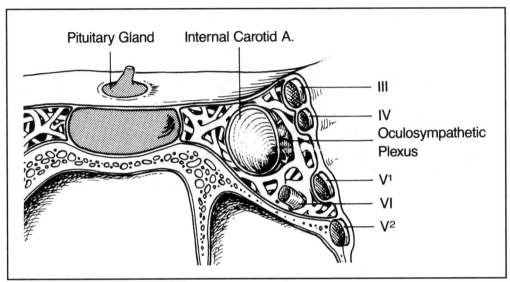

Figure 7-1. Coronal view of the left cavernous sinus and its contents.

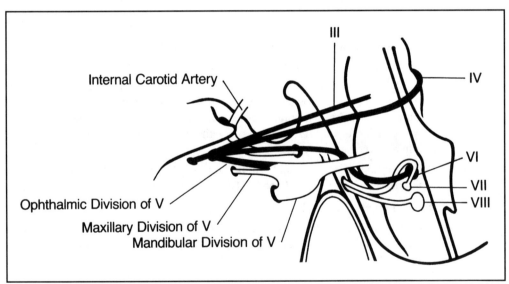

Figure 7-2. Lateral schematic view of the left cavernous sinus; cranial nerves that traverse the sinus are highlighted in black.

III.   Causes of cavernous sinus syndrome producing painful ophthalmoplegia

    A.   Trauma

    B.   Vascular

        1.   Intracavernous carotid artery aneurysm

        2.   Posterior cerebral artery aneurysm

        3.   Carotid-cavernous fistula

        4.   Carotid-cavernous sinus thrombosis

C. Neoplasm
    1. Primary intracranial tumor
       a. Pituitary adenoma
       b. Meningioma
       c. Craniopharyngioma
       d. Sarcoma
       e. Neurofibroma
       f. Gasserian ganglion neuroma
       g. Epidermoid
       h. Hemangioma/hemangiopericytoma
       i. Eosinophilic granuloma
    2. Primary cranial tumor
       a. Chordoma
       b. Chondroma
       c. Giant cell tumor
    3. Local metastases
       a. Nasopharyngeal tumor
       b. Cylindroma
       c. Adamantinoma
       d. Squamous cell carcinoma
    4. Distant metastases
       a. Lymphoma
       b. Multiple myeloma
       c. Carcinomatous metastases

D. Inflammation
    1. Bacterial: sinusitis, mucocele, periostitis
    2. Viral: herpes zoster
    3. Fungal: mucormycosis
    4. Spirochetal: Treponema pallidum
    5. Mycobacterial: Mycobacterium tuberculosis
    6. Unknown cause: sarcoidosis, Wegener's granulomatosis, Tolosa-Hunt syndrome

IV. Of the more common causes of cavernous sinus syndrome, these points deserve emphasis:

A. Intracavernous carotid artery aneurysm
    1. Typically produces slowly progressive, unilateral ophthalmoplegia
    2. May become painful
    3. Rarely rupture, but this occurrence produces a carotid-cavernous fistula

B. Carotid-cavernous fistula
    1. Due to direct communication between intracavernous carotid artery and cavernous sinus
    2. High-flow, high-pressure fistula
    3. Most common cause is head trauma
    4. Clinical picture: chemosis, proptosis, ocular motor nerve palsies, bruit, retinopathy, increased intraocular pressure

C. Dural-cavernous fistula
1. Due to communication of dural branches of internal or external carotid arteries and cavernous sinus or vessels in region of sinus
2. Low-flow, low-pressure fistula
3. Most commonly occur spontaneously
4. More subtle clinical picture: don't be fooled into treating these patients for "red eye"
5. A minority of patients may develop cortical venous drainage of their fistula, with increased risk of intracerebral hemorrhage or cerebral venous infarction. Suggestive clinical signs are bilateral orbital congestion and postauricular bruit. Workup: magnetic resonance imaging (MRI), magnetic resonance angiography (MRA), magnetic resonance venography (MRV), cerebral angiography
6. On occasion, fistula flow is directed posteriorly, causing chronic ocular motor cranial nerve palsies without orbital congestive signs ("white-eyed shunt")

D. Nasopharyngeal carcinoma
1. Two to three times more common in males
2. Predilection for Asian patients
3. Varied clinical presentation
    a. Nasal obstruction
    b. Rhinorrhea
    c. Epistaxis
    d. Otitis media
    e. Proptosis
    f. Ipsilateral dry eye
4. Ninety-five percent of patients with nasopharyngeal carcinoma have VI nerve paresis at some time during clinical course
5. Radiologic study of choice: cranial magnetic resonance scanning with attention to subcranial soft tissue in region of nasopharynx
6. Pharyngoscopy and biopsies of the nasopharynx if clinical suspicion high

E. Two aspects of neoplastic involvement of the parasellar region require particular attention
1. Mode of onset and clinical course do not prognosticate the type of lesion (ie, neoplastic disease may have an acute clinical presentation as well as an expected insidious course)
2. High-dose corticosteroid therapy may initially improve signs and symptoms due to neoplasm

F. Tolosa-Hunt syndrome
1. Painful ophthalmoplegia due to granulomatous inflammation occurring in the cavernous sinus
2. Spontaneous remissions may occur after days or weeks
3. Recurring attacks may occur at intervals of months or years
4. Systemic steroids usually lead to marked improvement of signs and symptoms within 48 hours
5. Categorically, diagnosis of exclusion and patients with this diagnosis require careful follow-up

V.   Imitators of cavernous sinus syndrome

A.   Myasthenia

B.   Ocular dysthyroidism

C.   Orbital disease: inflammation, infection, neoplasm, trauma

D.   Diabetic ophthalmoplegia

1.   Typically acute, often painful, mononeuropathy with full recovery within 3 months

2.   Less frequent occurrence of simultaneous paralysis of multiple ocular motor nerves. Often painful, recurrent, and not responsive to steroid therapy

E.   Giant cell arteritis

1.   Single or multiple ocular motor nerve palsies

2.   Produces ischemic necrosis of extraocular muscles

F.   Botulism

1.   Occurs in six forms: food-borne, wound, infantile, infant, hidden, inadvertent

2.   Ophthalmologic findings include dilated, poorly reactive pupils, ptosis, and ophthalmoplegia

3.   Affected individuals have nausea, vomiting, associated with facial, pharyngeal, and generalized proximal weakness, and no sensory deficits

4.   Botulinum toxin is the most potent poison known

5.   Causes cholinergic blockage by preventing release of acetylcholine at neuromuscular junction

G.   Miller Fisher syndrome

1.   Bulbar variant of Guillain-Barré syndrome, characterized by triad of ataxia, areflexia, ophthalmoplegia

2.   In evolution, this cranial polyneuropathy may mimic unilateral or bilateral ocular motor cranial nerve palsies, but usually progresses to a virtually total ophthalmoplegia with involvement of pupils and accommodation

3.   Patients may also have facial diplegia, respiratory and swallowing difficulties, and confusion

4.   Often follows gastroenteritis from Campylobacter jejuni infection

5.   Over 90% of patients have antibodies to the ganglioside GQ1b, which cross-reacts with ganglioside structure in wall of C. jejuni

6.   Anti GQ1b antibodies have been shown to damage the motor nerve terminal by a complement-mediated mechanism, possibly targeting neuronal membrane of presynaptic Schwann cells

7.   Bickerstaff's brainstem encephalitis is a closely related condition with alterations in consciousness and long tract signs seen in addition to ophthalmoplegia and ataxia

8.   Typically benign and self-limited

9.   If needed, treatment includes plasmapheresis and IV immunoglobulin (Ig)

VI.   Ocular neuromyotonia

A.   Patient reports episodic diplopia or oscillopsia

B.   Failure of extraocular muscles to "relax" following sustained, eccentric gaze

C.   Previous history of invasive pituitary adenoma or other intracranial tumors treated with radiation therapy

D.   Due to episodic, involuntary discharge of ocular motor nerves producing sustained and inappropriate contraction of their respective ocular muscles

E.   Treatment: carbamazepine, phenytoin

BIBLIOGRAPHY

Chapters

Parkinson D. Anatomy of the cavernous sinus. In: Smith JL, ed. *Neuro-Ophthalmology*. Vol 6. St Louis, Mo: CV Mosby; 1972:73-101.

Schatz NJ, Farmer P. Tolosa-Hunt syndrome: the pathology of painful ophthalmoplegia. In: Smith JL, ed. *Neuro-Ophthalmology*. Vol 6. St Louis, Mo: CV Mosby; 1972:102-112.

Articles

Acieino M, Trobe JD, Cornbluth WT, Gebarski SS. Painful oculomotor palsy caused by posterior-draining dural carotid cavernous fistulas. *Arch Ophthalmol*. 1995;113:1045-1049.

Barricks ME, Traviesa DB, Glaser JS, et al. Ophthalmoplegia in giant cell arteries. *Brain*. 1977;100:209-221.

Cherrington M: Botulism: update and review. *Sem Neurol*. 2004;24:155-163.

Chiba A, Kusonoki S, Obata H, Machinumi R, Kanazana I. Serum anti-GQ1b antibody is associated with ophthalmoplegia in Miller Fisher syndrome and Guillain-Barré syndrome: clinical and immunohistochemical studies. *Neurology*. 1993;43:1911-1917.

Fisher CM. An unusual variant of acute idiopathic polyneuritis (syndrome of ophthalmoplegia, ataxia, areflexia). *N Engl J Med*. 1956;255:57-65.

Harris FS, Rhoton AL. Anatomy of the cavernous sinus. A microsurgical study. *J Neurosurg*. 1976;45:169-180.

Kline LB, Hoyt WF. The Tolosa-Hunt syndrome. *J Neurol Neurosurg Psychiatry*. 2001;71:577-582.

Newton TH, Hoyt WF. Dural arteriovenous shunts in the region of the cavernous sinus. *Neuroradiology*. 1970;1:71-81.

Overell JR, Willison HJ. Recent developments in Miller Fisher syndrome and related disorders. *Curr Opin Neurol*. 2005;18:562-566.

Plant GT. Putting ocular neuromyotonia in context. *J Neuroophthalmol*. 2006;26:241-243.

Sanders MD, Hoyt WF. Hypoxic ocular sequelae of carotid-cavernous fistulae. *Br J Ophthalmol*. 1969;53:82-97.

Sergott RC, Grossman RI, Savino PJ, Bosley TM, Schatz NJ. The syndrome of paradoxical worsening of dural-cavernous sinus arteriovenous malformations. *Ophthalmology*. 1987;94:205-221.

Shults WT, Hoyt WF, Behrens MM, et al. Ocular neuromyotonia. *Arch Ophthalmol*. 1986;104:1028-1034.

Smith JL, Taxdal DSR. Painful ophthalmoplegia: the Tolosa-Hunt syndrome. *Am J Ophthalmol*. 1966;61:1466-1472.

Stiebel-Kalish H, Setton A, Berenstein A, et al. Bilateral orbital signs predict cortical venous drainage in cavernous sinus dural AVMs. *Neurology*. 2002;58:1521-1524.

Chapter 8

The Pupil

Lanning B. Kline, MD

I.   **Anatomical considerations**

   A.   Sphincter muscle of the iris

   1.   Innervated by parasympathetic fibers originating in the Edinger-Westphal (EW) nucleus, which forms part of the oculomotor nuclear complex in the midbrain

   2.   Input that excites the EW nucleus

   a.   Light reflex (Figure 8-1)

   i.   Afferent neurons from retinal ganglion cells to the pretectal area; intercalated neurons from the pretectal complex to EW nuclei; parasympathetic outflow with the oculomotor nerve to the ciliary ganglion and then to the iris sphincter muscle

   ii.   Monocular light information is carried by the optic nerve to the chiasm, where approximately half the fibers decussate to the contralateral optic tract, and half the fibers continue in the ipsilateral optic tract

   iii.   Approximately two thirds of the way along the optic tract, some of the axons leave the tract, enter the brachium of the superior colliculus, and synapse in the pretectal region

   iv.   The information is then passed forward via the intercalated neurons to the EW nuclei bilaterally

   v.   The pupillomotor information travels with the III nerve and through the superior orbital fissure with the inferior division

   vi.   Thus, light information received by one eye is transmitted to both pupils equally

   b.   Near synkinesis (Figure 8-2)

   i.   The peristriate cortex (area 19), at the upper end of the calcarine fissure, may be the origin of near synkinesis

   ii.   Near synkinesis triad

   a.   Convergence of eyes

   b.   Accommodation of the lenses

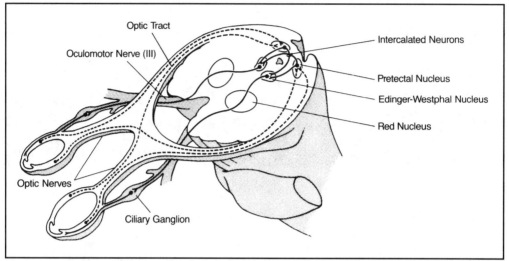

Figure 8-1. Pathway of the pupillary light reflex. (Adapted from Miller NR. *Walsh and Hoyt's Clinical Neuro-Ophthalmology.* 4th ed. Vol 2. Baltimore, Md: Williams & Wilkins; 1985:421.)

      c.   Miosis of the pupils

    iii.   The near synkinesis pathway is more ventrally located than the pretectal afferent limb of the light reflex. This separation of the "near" from "light" reflexes may be the anatomical basis for some instances of light-near dissociation of the pupils (eg, Argyll Robertson pupils, dorsal midbrain syndrome)

    iv.   The final pathway is the oculomotor nerve, ciliary ganglion, and the short posterior ciliary nerves. The ratio of ciliary ganglion cells that innervate the ciliary muscle vs cells related to iris sphincter is approximately 30:1

    3.   Input that inhibits EW nucleus

        a.   Cortical: dilated pupils during epileptic seizures

        b.   Spinal-reticular: states of arousal, excitement

        c.   Sleep, coma: inhibitory influences decline and pupils are miotic

  B.   Dilator muscle of the iris

    1.   Innervated by sympathetic fibers

    2.   Three neuron pathways (Figure 8-3):

        a.   First-order neuron originates in posterior hypothalamus and courses down through the brainstem to the C8-T2 level of the cord (ciliospinal center of Budge)

        b.   Second-order (preganglionic) neurons leave the cord, enter the paravertebral sympathetic chain, and terminate in the superior cervical ganglion at the base of the skull

        c.   Third-order (postganglionic) neuron fibers intended for the pupil and Muller's muscle ascend the internal carotid artery to enter the skull, join the ophthalmic nerve in the cavernous sinus, and then to the orbit through the superior orbital fissure; the sudomotor and vasomotor fibers to the face travel with the external carotid artery

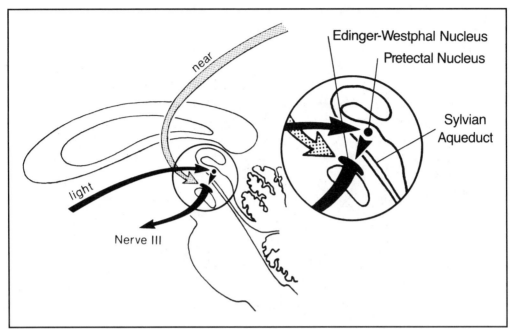

Figure 8-2. Illustration of a more ventral course of near response input (hatched arrow) to EW nucleus compared to light response input (solid arrow).

II. Normal pupillary phenomena

A. Physiologic anisocoria
1. Approximately 20% of the general population have clearly perceptible (generally less than 0.5 mm) anisocoria. The degree of anisocoria can vary from day to day and even switch sides

B. Pupillary unrest
1. During distance fixation and with constant, moderate, ambient illumination, the pupils will be noted to have bilaterally, symmetrically, nonrhythmical unrest or variation in size, usually less than 1 mm in amplitude of variation. This is termed hippus

C. Near synkinesis
1. With sufficient ambient illumination to allow visualization in the pupils, the patient is asked to shift fixation from the distant object to a near point, preferably the patient's own forefinger. Equal miosis of both pupils will be noted
2. After shifting fixation back to the distant object and maintaining the same ambient illumination, a bright light is placed before one or both eyes and the miosis of the light reflex is noted and compared to the "near" miosis. The "light" miosis will be equal to or greater than the "near" miosis
3. If a patient demonstrates normal reactions of the pupil to light, there is usually no clinical observation to be gained by testing the near response

D. Psychosensory reflex
1. While maintaining constant "near" and "light" stimuli, the examiner observes pupillary size with the use of a "startle" stimulus, such as a loud noise or pain

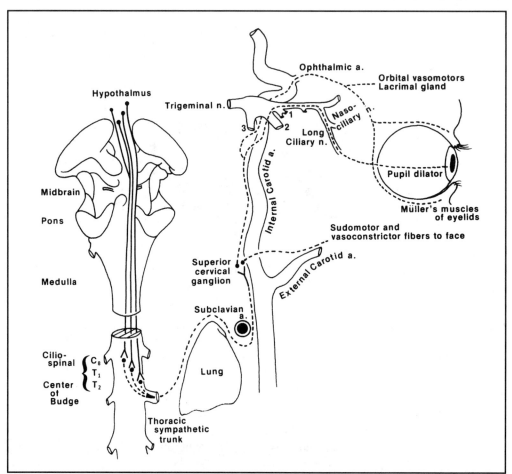

Figure 8-3. Diagram of oculosympathetic pathway. (Reprinted with permission from Slomovits TL, Glaser JS, The Pupils and Accommodation in *Duane's Clinical Ophthalmology* Vol 2, Tasman W, Jaeger E, eds. Lippincott Williams & Wilkins, 1994.)

    2. The pupils will dilate due to two neural mechanisms
       a. Active sympathetic discharges (stimulate iris dilator muscle)
       b. Inhibition of ocular motor nuclei (relaxation of iris sphincter muscle)
    3. The psychosensory reflex is helpful when demonstrating Horner's syndrome
  E. Direct pupillary light reflex
    1. By having the subject fixate on a distant object (thereby obviating the miosis associated with accommodation) and the ambient illumination moderately subdued, the direct pupillary response is noted when a bright light is placed before one eye
    2. The pupil constricts briskly, with a subsequent slow dilation to an intermediate size, followed by a state of pupillary unrest (hippus)
    3. The normalcy of the briskness and the latency of the initial response can be evaluated by clinical experience but will be further evaluated by comparison with the fellow eye during the direct light reflex test as well as during the swinging flashlight test (see next page)

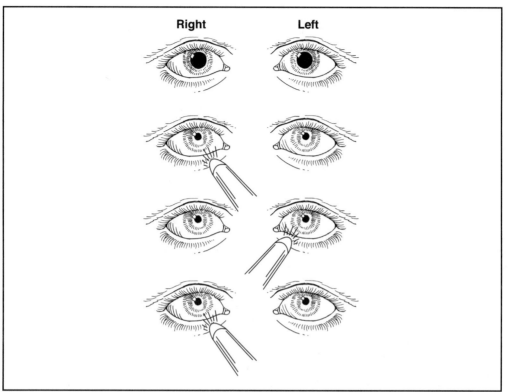

Figure 8-4. Normal response to swinging flashlight test with no change in size of pupils.

4.   The amplitudes of the initial constriction and subsequent redilation (pupillary escape) depend upon the ambient illumination and the relative brightness of the test light. These amplitudes are also subject to marked individual variation and are best evaluated by comparison with the fellow eye during the swinging flashlight test

F.   Consensual pupillary reflex
  1.   Because of the equal distribution (to both III nerves) of the photic information provided by one eye, the fellow pupil will behave in the same manner described above for the direct light reflex

G.   Swinging flashlight test (Figure 8-4)
  1.   While maintaining the same test conditions described in testing the direct pupillary light reflex, the examiner projects the light on (for example) the right eye and allows the right to go through the phase of initial constriction to a minimum size and subsequent escape to an intermediate size
  2.   At this point, the examiner quickly swings the light to the left eye, which will begin at the intermediate size and go through the phase of initial constriction to a minimum size and subsequent escape to an intermediate size
  3.   As soon as the left pupil redilates to the intermediate size, the light is swung to the right eye and a mental note made of the intermediate (starting) size, the latency and briskness of the response, the minimum size, the latency and briskness of the redilation of the intermediate size

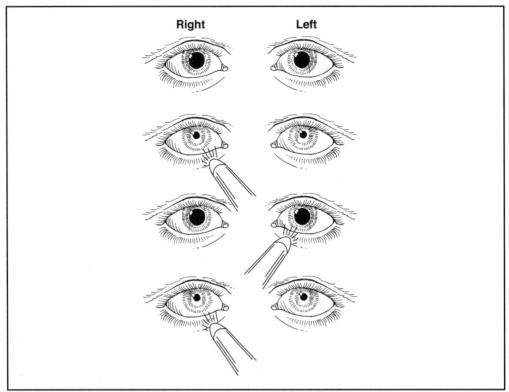

Figure 8-5. Afferent pupillary defect in the left eye using a swinging flashlight test. The pupils constrict when the light is shined in the right eye; however, when the flashlight is swung back to the left eye, both pupils dilate.

      4.   These characteristics will be exactly the same in both eyes as the light is alternately swung to each eye

      5.   Key points in proper testing:

          a.   A bright hand light in a darkened room is essential

          b.   The patient should fix on a distant object

          c.   The light should cross from one eye to the other fairly rapidly (across the bridge of the nose) and remain 3 to 5 seconds on each eye to allow pupillary stabilization

III.   Abnormal pupillary states

    A.   Afferent pupillary defect (Marcus Gunn pupil) (Figure 8-5)

      1.   During the swinging flashlight test, if the amount of light information transmitted from one eye is less than that carried from the fellow eye, the following phenomenon may be noted when the light is swung from the normal eye to the defective eye

          a.   Immediate dilation of the pupil, instead of normal initial constriction (3 to 4+ Marcus Gunn pupil)

          b.   No change in pupil size initially, followed by dilation of the pupils (1 to 2+ Marcus Gunn pupil)

c. Initial constriction, but greater escape to a larger intermediate size than when the light is swung back to the normal eye (trace Marcus Gunn pupil)

2. When the light is swung back to the normal eye, the pupil demonstrates the normal pattern of brisk constriction (of short latency) with subsequent escape to an intermediate size

3. Optic neuropathy (must be unilateral or markedly asymmetric) will usually present with a significant Marcus Gunn pupil

4. Afferent pupillary defect can be quantified using neutral density filters (0.3, 0.6, 0.9 log unit values). Appropriate amount of filter is placed before normal eye to neutralize the afferent pupillary defect so that pupils constrict equally and reach the same final resting size

5. Opacities of the ocular media (corneal scar, cataract, vitreous hemorrhage) will not cause a Marcus Gunn pupillary phenomenon if a strong enough flashlight is used

6. Maculopathy, or amblyopic "lazy eye," will not cause a Marcus Gunn phenomenon unless very extensive (less than 20/200 acuity) and then it will only be a 1+ phenomenon, compared to a 3 to 4+ if the 20/200 acuity was due to an optic neuropathy

7. Extensive retinal damage will cause a significant Marcus Gunn phenomenon

8. Amaurotic pupil: the maximum Marcus Gunn pupil imaginable; seen in patients with "blind eye"

9. There is no such thing as "bilateral" Marcus Gunn pupils; there may be bilaterally reduced direct response of the pupils to light, resulting in "light-near" dissociation, but the Marcus Gunn phenomenon requires asymmetry of the afferent light transmission

10. Isolated, unilateral optic neuropathy does not cause the ipsilateral pupil to be larger; the pupils remain the same size because of the consensual reflex. Unilateral amaurotic mydriasis does not exist

11. Detection of the afferent pupillary defect requires only one "working" pupil. If one pupil is mechanically or pharmacologically nonreactive, one can simply perform a swinging flashlight test observing the reactive pupil. If the abnormal eye is the eye with a fixed pupil, then the pupil of the normal eye will constrict briskly when the light is shined directly in it and will dilate when the light is shined in the opposite eye. If the abnormal eye is the eye with the reactive pupil, then the pupil will constrict when light is shined in the opposite eye and will dilate when light is shined directly in it

12. Rarely, an afferent pupillary defect occurs without visual acuity loss or a visual field defect. Due to lesion involving pupillomotor fibers traversing brachium of superior colliculus while sparing visual fibers in the optic tract

B. Adie's tonic pupil
1. Idiopathic, benign cause of internal ophthalmoplegia
2. Eighty percent unilateral initially; tends to become bilateral at a rate of 4% per year
3. Female predilection (70% vs 30%)
4. Young adults: 20 to 40 years of age

5.   Dilated pupil with poor to absent light reaction

6.   Slow constriction to prolonged near-effort and slow redilation (tonic response) after near effort

7.   Most patients initially have accommodative paresis, which usually resolves over several months

8.   Primary finding of segmental palsy of iris sphincter muscle

9.   Adie's pupil frequently (80% of cases) demonstrates cholinergic supersensitivity to weak pilocarpine solutions (0.125% or 0.10%)

10. Etiology in most cases is unknown. Lesion causing Adie's pupil located in the ciliary ganglion or short posterior ciliary nerves; aberrant regeneration of more numerous fibers innervating the ciliary muscle (97%) into those subserving the iris sphincter muscle (3%)

11. Adie's syndrome: pupillary abnormalities occurring in a patient with associated diminished deep tendon reflexes

C.   Argyll Robertson pupils

1.   Miotic, irregular pupils

2.   Absence of pupillary light response associated with normal anterior visual pathway function

3.   Brisk pupillary constriction to near stimuli

4.   Poor dilation in the dark and in response to mydriatic agents

5.   Condition is usually bilateral, but is often asymmetric and may be unilateral

6.   Etiology: major consideration is neurosyphilis. Other reported causes include diabetes mellitus, chronic alcoholism, multiple sclerosis, sarcoidosis

7.   Site of lesion: most likely in the region of the Sylvian aqueduct in the rostral midbrain interfering with the light reflex fibers and supranuclear inhibitory fibers as they approach the EW nuclei. More ventrally located fibers for near response are spared (see Figure 8-2)

D.   Light-near dissociation of the pupils

1.   Better pupillary response to "near" than to "light"

2.   Differential diagnosis

a.   Optic neuropathy or severe retinopathy (probably most common cause)

b.   Adie's tonic pupil

c.   Argyll Robertson pupils

d.   Dorsal midbrain syndrome

e.   Aberrant regeneration of III nerve; defective response to light with aberrent hook-up of medial rectus fibers to the pupillary fibers, resulting in pupillary constriction during adduction

f.   Miscellaneous causes: amyloidosis, diabetes, Dejerine-Sottas, Charcot-Marie-Tooth

E.   The pupils of coma

1.   Hutchinson pupil

a.   Comatose patient with unilaterally dilated, poorly reactive pupil

b.   Probably due to ipsilateral, expanding, intracranial, supratentorial mass (eg, tumor, subdural hematoma) that is causing downward displacement of hippocampal gyrus and uncal herniation across the tentorial edge with entrapment of the III nerve (see Figure 5-4)

        c.   The pupillomotor fibers travel in the peripheral portion of the III nerve (near the perineurium) and are subject to early damage from compression

    2.   Miosis

        a.   During the early stages of coma, the cortical inhibitory input to the EW nucleus is diminished and the pupils are small but reactive to light

        b.   Remember pharmacologic miosis

            i.   Morphine

            ii.   Pilocarpine: if the patient is being incidentally treated for glaucoma

F.   The pupils of hospital personnel (pharmacologic blockade)

    1.   Unilaterally dilated, fixed pupil

    2.   Due to inadvertent contact with mydriatic agent, most commonly atropine

G.   Traumatic pupil

    1.   Contusion injury of the eye may cause miosis or mydriasis

    2.   Miosis may be due to sphincter spasm seen with iritis

    3.   Mydriasis may be due to contusion injury (or actual rupture) of the iris sphincter muscle

        a.   Irregular pupil

        b.   Poorly responsive to 1% pilocarpine

H.   Pharmacologic differentiation of the causes of a fixed, dilated pupil

    1.   The patient is tested first with 0.1% pilocarpine, then, if necessary, 1% pilocarpine

    2.   If the pupil constricts to 0.1% pilocarpine, then the patient has Adie's pupil; if there is no response to 0. 1% pilocarpine, then proceed to 1%

    3.   If 1% pilocarpine constricts the involved pupil, then the patient may have a III nerve paresis

    4.   If 1% pilocarpine fails to constrict the involved pupil, or does so poorly, the patient has either pharmacologic blockade or a traumatic pupil

I.   Horner's syndrome (oculosympathetic paralysis)

    1.   Three neuron pathways (see Figure 8-3)

    2.   Clinical signs:

        a.   Miosis of the affected pupil, which is more marked in dim illumination (evoking dilation) than in bright illumination

        b.   Ptosis of the upper lid; usually 2 to 3 mm

        c.   Upside-down ptosis of the low lid (due to paresis of inferior tarsal muscle), causing the lower lid to rest 1 to 2 mm higher on the affected side

        d.   Apparent enophthalmos due to narrow palpebral fissure

        e.   Anhydrosis of the affected side of the face. This occurs only if the lesion involves the sympathetic pathway proximal to the bifurcation of the common carotid artery, since the sudomotor fibers travel with the external carotid artery

        f.   Heterochromia of the affected iris. Characteristic of congenital Horner's with the affected eye having a lighter color

g.   Transient findings

      i.   Dilated conjunctival and facial vessels

      ii.   Decreased intraocular pressure

      iii.   Increased accommodation

3.   Diagnostic steps in suspected Horner's syndrome

    a.   Amount of anisocoria should increase in dim vs bright illumination. If this step seems inconclusive, then proceed to cocaine test

    b.   Cocaine test

      i.   Cocaine (4% to 10%) eyedrops creating sympathomimetic effect by blocking the receptors of norepinephrine at the myoneural junction, thereby prolonging the action of norepinephrine upon the dilator muscle

      ii.   Therefore, cocaine requires release of norepinephrine at the myoneural junction by a normal functioning oculosympathetic pathway

      iii.   Cocaine drops result in dilation of the normal pupil

      iv.   If there is a lesion involving any of the three neurons, pupillary inequality will increase, and the presence of Horner's syndrome is confirmed

      v.   Anisocoria of 1 mm or more following instillation of cocaine drops signifies Horner's syndrome

    c.   Paredrine test

      i.   Paredrine (1% hydroxyamphetamine) eyedrops create a sympathomimetic effect by causing release of ñorepinephrine from the nerve endings at the myoneural junction, thereby stimulating the dilator muscle

      ii.   Paredrine requires that the third-order (postganglionic) neuron be intact and have normal axoplasmic activity, including formation and transfer of norepinephrine to the nerve ending at the myoneural junction

      iii.   Paredrine drops result in dilation of the normal pupil

      iv.   If there is a lesion of the third-order neuron, there will be subnormal dilation of the pupil by Paredrine

      v.   Pupillary dilation to Paredrine drops will be normal if the Horner's syndrome is due to lesions of the first- or second-order neurons

    d.   Therefore, cocaine serves to confirm the presence of Horner's syndrome and Paredrine serves to identify Horner's due to lesions of the third-order neuron

    e.   Aproclonidine drops (1% or 0.5%) may also help in establishing diagnosis of Horner's syndrome

      i.   Causes reversal of anisocoria with dilation of affected pupil and no effect on normal pupillary size

      ii.   Possibly due to denervation hypersensitivity of α-1 receptor of pupillary dilator muscle ipsilateral to the Horner's syndrome

    f.   Beware of pseudo-Horner's syndrome: ipsilateral ptosis and miosis of unrelated cause

4. Differentiation of causes of Horner's syndrome
    a. First-order neuron lesion (brainstem and spinal cord)
        i. Cerebrovascular accident (Wallenberg's syndrome)
        ii. Neck trauma
        iii. Neoplasm
        iv. Demyelinating disease
        v. Syringomyelia
    b. Second-order neuron lesion (preganglionic)
        i. Chest lesions: occult carcinoma of the lung apex (Pancoast's tumor), mediastinal mass, cervical rib
        ii. Neck lesions: trauma, abscess, thyroid neoplasm, lymphadenopathy
        iii. Surgery: thyroidectomy, radical neck surgery, carotid angiography (direct carotid puncture)
    c. Third-order neuron lesion (postganglionic)
        i. Lesion may be extracranial (similar etiologies as listed for second-order neuron neck lesions) or cause may be intracranial
        ii. Migraine variants: cluster headaches, Raeder's paratrigeminal neuralgia
        iii. Complicated otitis media
        iv. Cavernous sinus/superior orbital fissure lesion
        v. Internal carotid artery dissection
        vi. Carotid-cavernous fistula
        vii. Nasopharyngeal carcinoma
5. Horner's syndrome in children
    a. Horner's syndrome present at birth usually benign and associated with heterochromia
    b. Usually idiopathic (30% to 70%); may be associated with birth trauma (brachial plexus injury); rarely due to intrauterine neuroblastoma
    c. Second-order neuron lesion (eg, chest tumor) often behaves pharmacologically like third-order neuron lesion (fails to dilate to hydroxyamphetamine). Probably due to transsynaptic degeneration of preganglionic neuron
    d. Acquired Horner's syndrome in first 5 years of life is a more ominous occurrence; often due to neuroblastoma involving sympathetic chain in chest or neck
    e. In both congenital and acquired Horner's syndrome, a pediatric evaluation is warranted

IV. **Evaluation of a patient with anisocoria (Figure 8-6)**

V. **Rare pupillary disorders**
    A. Benign episodic pupillary dilatation ("springing pupil")
        1. Young, healthy adults
        2. Variable history of migraine
        3. Characteristics:

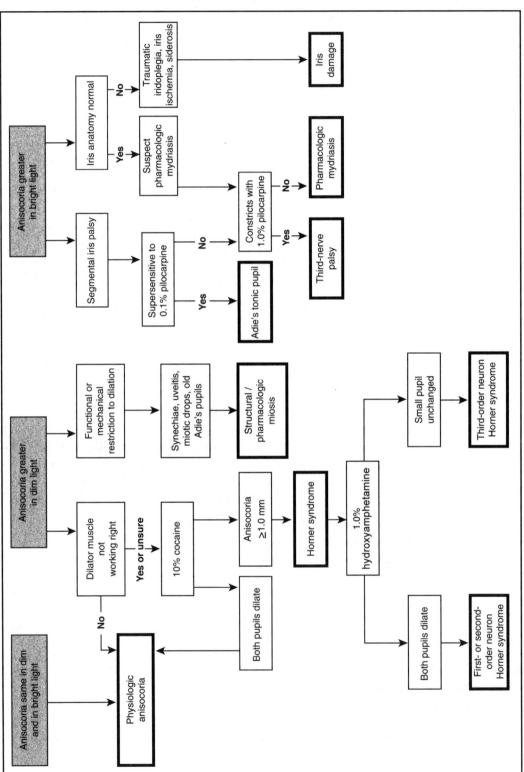

Figure 8-6. Flowchart for evaluation of anisocoria. (Reproduced, with permission, from Kline LB, *Basic and Clinical Science Course: Section 5*, Ameri-

    a.   One pupil widely dilated for minutes to hours
    b.   Mild blurring of vision
    c.   May have associated periocular discomfort
    d.   Headache occurring following episode
  4. Must exclude accidental pharmacologic blockade
  5. Uniformly benign condition

B. Tadpole pupils
  1. Sectoral pupillary dilation lasting for a few minutes, then returning to normal
  2. Occurs multiple times per day for several days or a week and then disappears
  3. Unusual periocular sensation draws attention to the pupil
  4. Patient may have history of migraine
  5. Possibly due to segmental spasm of iris dilator muscle
  6. Benign condition

C. Midbrain corectopia
  1. Eccentric or oval pupil seen in patients with rostral midbrain disease
  2. Thought to be due to selective inhibition of iris sphincter tone
  3. Oval pupils may also be seen with midbrain dysfunction due to extrinsic compression from shift of midline supratentorial structures

D. Paradoxical pupils
  1. Pupillary constriction in darkness
  2. Initially felt to be a sign of retinal disease (congenital stationary night blindness, congenital achromatopsia)
  3. More recently observed in anomalies of optic nerve development (optic nerve coloboma, optic nerve hypoplasia), congenital nystagmus, and a variety of retinal disorders (retinitis pigmentosa, Best's disease, macular dystrophy, albinism)
  4. Mechanism of phenomenon unknown

BIBLIOGRAPHY

Books

Lowenfeld IE. *The Pupil: Anatomy, Physiology and Clinical Applications*. Boston, Mass: Butterworth-Heinemann; 1999.

Chapters

Burde RM, Savino PJ, Trobe JD. *Clinical Decisions in Neuro-Ophthalmology*. 3rd ed. St Louis, Mo: Mosby; 2002:246-271.

Kardon RH. Anatomy and physiology of the autonomic nervous system. In: Miller NR, Newman NJ, eds. *Walsh and Hoyt's Clinical Neuro-Ophthalmology*. 6th ed. Vol 1. Philadelphia, Pa: Lippincott Williams & Wilkins; 2005:649-714.

Slamovits TL, Glaser JS. The pupils and accommodation. In: Glaser JS. *Neuro-Ophthalmology*. 3rd ed. Philadelphia, Pa: Lippincott Williams & Wilkins; 1999:527-552.

Articles

Cremer SA, Thompson HS, Digre KB, Kardon RH. Hydroxyamphetamine mydriasis in Horner's syndrome. *Am J Ophthalmol*. 1990;110:66-70.

Forman S, Behrens MM, Odel JG, et al. Relative afferent pupillary defect with normal visual function. *Arch Ophthalmol*. 1990;108:1074-1075.

Frank JW, Kushner BJ, France TD. Paradoxic pupillary phenomena. *Arch Ophthalmol*. 1988;106:1564-1566.

Freedman KA, Brown SM. Topical aproclonidine in the diagnosis of suspected Horner syndrome. *J Neuroophthalmol*. 2005;25:83-85.

Jacobson DM. Benign episodic unilateral mydriasis: clinical characteristics. *Ophthalmology*. 1995;102:1623-1627.

Jeffery AR, Ellis FJ, Repka MX, Buncic JR. Pediatric Horner's syndrome. *Journal of the American Association for Pediatric Ophthalmology and Strabismus*. 1998;2:159-167.

Kardon RH, Denison CE, Brown C, Thompson HS. Critical evaluation of the cocaine test in the diagnosis of Horner's syndrome. *Arch Ophthalmol*. 1990;108:384-387.

Levitan P. Pupillary escape in disease of the retina or optic nerve. *Arch Ophthalmol*. 1959;62:768-779.

Loewenfeld IE. "Simple, central" anisocoria: a common condition, seldom recognized. *Transactions of the American Academy of Ophthalmology and Otolaryngology*. 1977;83:832-839.

Loewenfeld IE. The Argyll Robertson pupil, 1869-1969. A critical survey of the literature. *Surv Ophthalmol*. 1969;14:199-299.

Selhorst JB, Hoyt WF, Feinsod M, et al. Midbrain correctopia. *Arch Neurol*. 1976;33:193-195.

Thompson BM, Corbett JJ, Kline LB, et al. Pseudo-Horner's syndrome. *Arch Neurol*. 1982;39:108-111.

Thompson HS. Adie's syndrome: some new observations. *Trans Am Ophthalmol Soc*. 1977;75:587-626.

Thompson HS, Newsome DA, Lowenfeld IE. The fixed dilated pupil: sudden iridoplegia or mydriatic drops? A simple diagnostic test. *Arch Ophthalmol*. 1971;86:21-27.

Thompson HS, Pilley SEJ. Unequal pupils. A flow chart for sorting out the anisocorias. *Surv Ophthalmol*. 1976;21:45-48.

Thompson HS, Zackon DH, Czarnecki JSC. Tadpole-shaped pupils caused by segmental spasm of the iris dilator muscle. *Am J Ophthalmol*. 1983;96:467-472.

Chapter 9

The Swollen Optic Disc

Lanning B. Kline, MD

I. **Definitions**

　　A. Optic disc edema, swollen disc, "choked" disc: general terms used to describe the optic nerve head affected by a variety of local and systemic causes (Table 9-1)

　　B. Papilledema: edema of the optic discs due to increased intracranial pressure being transmitted to the optic nerves by the cerebrospinal fluid (CSF) in the subarachnoid space

II. **Pathophysiology of optic disc edema**

　　A. Axonal (axoplasmic) transport along ganglion cell axons that form the optic nerve occurs in anterograde (cell body to lateral geniculate nucleus) and retrograde (geniculate nucleus to cell body) direction

　　B.

Axonal Transport Type	*Motor Protein*
Anterograde	Kinesin
Fast: 50 to 400 mm/day	
Slow:	
Type a: 0.3 to 3 mm/day	
Type b: 2 to 8 mm/day	
Retrograde	Dynein
Fast: 200 to 400 mm/day	

　　C. Anterograde flow mainly involves transport of neurally synthesized proteins, while retrograde transport is concerned with movement of endosomes and lysosomes

　　D. Accumulation of axoplasmic flow, especially slow anterograde component, at the lamina cribrosa produces disc swelling and nerve fiber layer (NFL) opacification

　　E. In papilledema, increased perineural pressure results in damming of the axoplasmic transport. Other causes of interrupted axonal transport include inflammation (eg, papillitis) and ischemia (eg, ischemic optic neuropathy [ION])

　　F. Secondary associated phenomena include dilated retinal veins, exudates, hemorrhages, cotton-wool spots (microinfarcts of the NFL)

Table 9-1

CAUSES OF OPTIC DISC EDEMA

Ocular Disease
Uveitis
Hypotony
Vein occlusion

Disc Tumors
Hemangioma
Glioma
Metastatic

Metabolic
Dysthyroidism
Juvenile diabetes
Proliferative retinopathies

Vascular
Ischemic neuropathy
Arteritis, cranial
Arteritis, collagen

Inflammatory
Papillitis
Neuroretinitis
Papillophlebitis

Orbital Tumors
Perioptic meningioma
Glioma
Sheath "cysts"
Retrobulbar mass

Infiltrative
Lymphoma
Reticuloendothelial

Elevated Intracranial Pressure
Mass lesion
Pseudotumor cerebri
Hypertension

Systemic Disease
Anemia
Hypoxemia
Hypertension
Uremia

Modified from Glaser JS. *Neuro-Ophthalmology.* 3rd ed. Philadelphia, Pa: Lippincott Williams & Wilkins; 1999:138.

III. **Papilledema**

    A.   Ophthalmoscopic features

        1.   Bilateral disc edema (may be asymmetric; rarely unilateral)

        2.   Opacification of peripapillary NFL

        3.   Hyperemia of disc (superficial capillary telangiectasias)

        4.   Absent venous pulsations (if venous pulsations are present, then the CSF pressure is probably less than 200 mm of water, 20% of normal patients have absent venous pulsations; therefore, the phenomenon of venous pulsations is helpful only if present)

        5.   Splinter hemorrhages (ie, hemorrhages within the NFL)

        6.   Exudates

        7.   Cotton-wool spots

        8.   Haziness of the retinal vessels at the disc margins due to swelling of the NFL in which the retinal vessels course

        9.   Circumferential retinal folds (Paton's lines) in peripapillary region

      10.   Obliterated central cup—usually a late finding in papilledema

    B.   Diagnosis of papilledema constitutes a medical emergency

        1.   Cranial computed tomography (CT) or magnetic resonance imaging (MRI) to rule out mass lesion

    2.   Magnetic resonance venography (MRV) also performed to exclude cerebral venous sinus thrombosis (see Chapter 9, IV, F)

    3.   If no mass is discovered and the ventricles are not dilated, CSF analysis to measure opening pressure and look carefully for infectious, inflammatory, or neoplastic cause

C.   Visual loss in chronic papilledema

    1.   Enlarged blind spots on visual field examination

    2.   Transient obscurations of vision, unilateral or bilateral "blacking out" or "graying out" of vision lasting 10 to 15 seconds and recurring many times per day; often precipitated by sudden changes in posture

    3.   Small, glistening hard exudates become apparent in the superficial disc substance ("pseudo-drusen"); may represent chronic axoplasmic stasis

    4.   Gradually, progressive visual field loss, usually beginning nasally and leading to generalized constriction

    5.   Chronic atrophic papilledema with eventual loss of central acuity

IV. Pseudotumor cerebri

A.   Diagnostic criteria

    1.   Awake and alert patient

    2.   Signs and symptoms of increased intracranial pressure (headache, nausea, vomiting, transient visual obstructions, papilledema, diplopia)

    3.   Absence of localizing findings on neurologic examination

    4.   Neuroimaging studies demonstrate normal ventricular system

    5.   Lumbar puncture reveals increased CSF pressure (>200 mm water in non-obese patient and >250 mm water in obese patient)

    6.   No other cause of increased intracranial pressure present

B.   In addition to papilledema, ophthalmologic findings may include:

    1.   VI nerve palsy (see VI_2 syndrome in Chapter 4)

    2.   Visual field changes (large blind spots, generalized constriction)

C.   Patients are frequently young adult, obese females who otherwise report a sense of well-being

D.   MRI may demonstrate:

    1.   Flattening of the posterior sclera

    2.   Enhancement of the prelaminar optic nerve

    3.   Distention of the perioptic subarachnoid space

    4.   Intraocular protrusion of the prelaminar optic nerve

    5.   Vertical tortuosity of the orbital optic nerve

    6.   Empty sella

E.   Management

    1.   Weight loss: as little as 6% reduction has beneficial effect

    2.   Medication: acetazolamide, furosemide, corticosteroids, analgesics

    3.   Optic nerve sheath decompression (see Chapter 20, V), neurosurgical shunting procedure (CSF diversion)

F.   Other settings associated with increased intracranial pressure in the absence of a CNS mass lesion:

1. Cerebral venous sinus thrombosis—detected with MRV
2. Variety of other systemic disorders (Table 9-2)
3. These settings lead to "secondary" pseudotumor cerebri syndromes

V. Optic neuritis

A. Primary inflammation of the optic nerve

B. Two clinical forms of optic neuritis:
1. Papillitis—intraocular form in which disc swelling is present
2. Retrobulbar neuritis—optic disc appears normal and inflammatory lesion along course of optic nerve is behind globe

C. Acute impairment of vision

D. Usually unilateral, although may be bilateral, especially in children

E. Occurs in young (14 to 45 years) adults; females outnumber males (5:1)

F. Pain: periocular, retrobulbar, tenderness of the globe, pain especially with eye movement

G. Afferent pupillary defect present if optic neuritis is unilateral

H. Visual field defects: usually central scotoma, but may be centrocecal or nerve fiber bundle defects

I. Cells in vitreous with papillitis

J. Chronological pattern of visual loss: rapid decrease in acuity during the first 2 or 3 days; stable level of decreased vision for 7 to 10 days, then gradual improvement of vision, frequently returning to normal level within 2 to 3 months

K. Uhthoff's symptom: dimming of vision in affected eye with elevation of body temperature (eg, exercise, hot shower, fever) with active or recurrent optic neuritis

L. Etiologies of optic neuritis
1. Idiopathic
2. Multiple sclerosis
3. Neuromyelitis optica ([NMO] Devic's syndrome)
    a. Bilateral optic neuritis associated with transverse myelitis
    b. Propensity for children and young adults
    c. Extensive, longitudinal spinal cord lesions spanning three or more vertebral segments
    d. Separate entity from multiple sclerosis
        i. Lack of paraventricular white matter lesions on MRI
        ii. Spinal fluid demonstrates inflammatory cells but no evidence of IgG synthesis
    e. Associated with IgG autoantibody (NMO-IgG)
    f. Less predictable course for good visual and neurologic recovery than multiple sclerosis
    g. Treatment: corticosteroids, immunosuppressive agents (eg, azathioprine), plasmapheresis
4. Viral infections: childhood (eg, mumps, measles, chicken pox), adult (eg, zoster)
5. Postviral syndrome

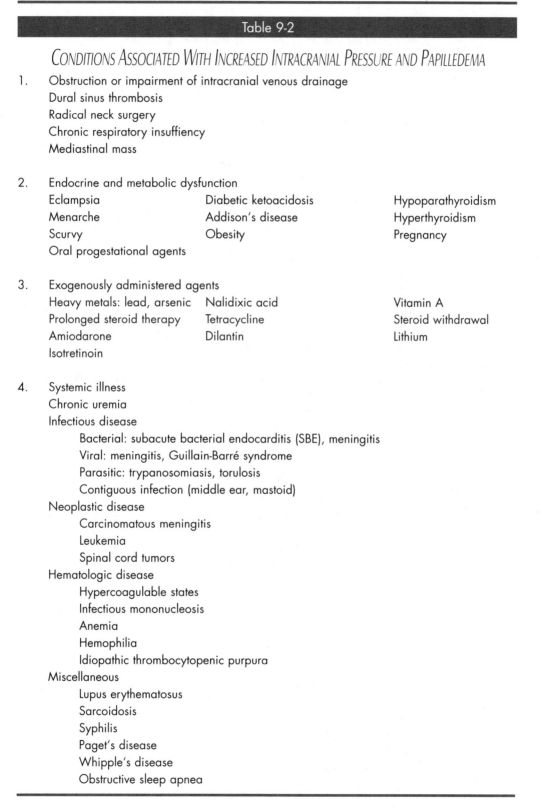

Table 9-2

CONDITIONS ASSOCIATED WITH INCREASED INTRACRANIAL PRESSURE AND PAPILLEDEMA

1. Obstruction or impairment of intracranial venous drainage
    Dural sinus thrombosis
    Radical neck surgery
    Chronic respiratory insuffiency
    Mediastinal mass

2. Endocrine and metabolic dysfunction

Eclampsia	Diabetic ketoacidosis	Hypoparathyroidism
Menarche	Addison's disease	Hyperthyroidism
Scurvy	Obesity	Pregnancy
Oral progestational agents		

3. Exogenously administered agents

Heavy metals: lead, arsenic	Nalidixic acid	Vitamin A
Prolonged steroid therapy	Tetracycline	Steroid withdrawal
Amiodarone	Dilantin	Lithium
Isotretinoin		

4. Systemic illness
    Chronic uremia
    Infectious disease
          Bacterial: subacute bacterial endocarditis (SBE), meningitis
          Viral: meningitis, Guillain-Barré syndrome
          Parasitic: trypanosomiasis, torulosis
          Contiguous infection (middle ear, mastoid)
    Neoplastic disease
          Carcinomatous meningitis
          Leukemia
          Spinal cord tumors
    Hematologic disease
          Hypercoagulable states
          Infectious mononucleosis
          Anemia
          Hemophilia
          Idiopathic thrombocytopenic purpura
    Miscellaneous
          Lupus erythematosus
          Sarcoidosis
          Syphilis
          Paget's disease
          Whipple's disease
          Obstructive sleep apnea

6.   Intraocular inflammation
7.   Contiguous inflammation (eg, meninges, orbit, sinuses)
8.   Systemic illness (eg, sarcoid, syphilis, tuberculosis)

M.   Optic Neuritis Treatment Trial (ONTT)
1.   Prospective, randomized study of 457 patients with optic neuritis
2.   Three treatment groups:
   a.   Oral prednisone (1 mg/kg/day) for 14 days
   b.   Intravenous methylprednisolone (1000 mg/day) for 3 days, followed by oral prednisone (1 mg/kg/day) for 11 days
   c.   Oral placebo for 14 days
3.   Fastest recovery for intravenous group, but at 1-year follow-up and thereafter no significant difference in visual recovery among three groups
4.   At 1-year follow-up 91% to 95% of patients in three groups regained acuity of 20/40 or better
5.   Patients treated with oral prednisone had significantly higher rates of new attacks of optic neuritis
6.   Group receiving intravenous regimen and having two or more typical demyelinating white matter lesions on MRI; had a significantly lower rate of developing multiple sclerosis within 2 years of follow-up than did the placebo or prednisone groups. However, this benefit was no longer measurable after 3 years of follow-up
7.   Visual prognosis for optic neuritis generally good. ONTT at 5-year follow-up:
   a.   20/25 or better: 87%
   b.   20/30 to 20/40: 7%
   c.   20/50 to 20/190: 3%
   d.   20/200 or worse: 3%
8.   Overall probability of developing clinically definite multiple sclerosis at 5 years=30%; 10 years=38%
9.   MRI findings are strongest predictor of developing clinically definite multiple sclerosis at 10-year follow-up:
   a.   No MRI lesions: 22%
   b.   One or more lesions: 56%
   c.   Greater number of lesions on MRI does not increase likelihood of developing multiple sclerosis
10. Combination of the following seen to substantially decrease likelihood of developing multiple sclerosis:
   a.   Severe optic disc edema
   b.   Visual acuity ≥20/40
   c.   Lack of periocular pain

N.   Controlled High-Risk Subjects Avonex Multiple Sclerosis Prevention Study (CHAMPS)
1.   Prospective, randomized study of 383 patients with first acute demyelinating event (optic neuritis, myelitis, brainstem, cerebellum) and at least two MRI white matter signal abnormalities

2. Treatment groups

    a. ONTT protocol IV/oral steroids (see Chapter 9, V, M, 2, b) followed by weekly intramuscular injection of 30 micrograms of interferon ß-1a (Avonex [Biogen Idec, Cambridge, Mass])

    b. ONTT protocol IV/oral steroids followed by weekly intramuscular injection of placebo

3. Results: 3-year follow-up

    a. Development of clinically definite multiple sclerosis significantly lower in interferon ß-1a group

    b. Reduction in volume of brain lesions in interferon ß-1a group

    c. Fewer new or enlarging lesions and fewer gadolinium enhancing lesions in interferon ß-1a group

    d. Trial terminated because of clear benefit of therapy over placebo

O. Early Treatment of Multiple Sclerosis (ETOMS) Study Group

1. Prospective, randomized, multicenter, double-blind study of 300 patients experiencing first episode of neurologic dysfunction suggesting multiple sclerosis within the previous 3 months and strongly suggestive brain MRI findings

2. Treatment groups

    a. Interferon ß-1a (Rebif [EMD Serono, Rockland, Mass]) 22 micrograms subcutaneously once per week

    b. Placebo injected subcutaneously once per week

3. Results: 2-year follow-up

    a. Fewer patients developed clinically definite multiple sclerosis (34%) vs the placebo group (45%) (p=0.047)

    b. For 30% of each group to convert to clinically definite multiple sclerosis (CDMS) required 569 days in treatment group vs 252 in placebo group (p=0.034)

    c. Annual relapse rate in treatment group was 0.33 vs 0.43 with placebo (p=0.045)

    d. Number and total volume of new T2-weighted MRI lesions lower in treatment group

P. Betaseron (Chiron, Emeryville, Calif) in newly emerging multiple sclerosis for initial treatment (BENEFIT) trial

1. Prospective, randomized, multicenter, double-blind study of 468 patients experiencing first clinical demyelinating event (monofocal or multifocal) and at least two brain MRI lesions

2. Treatment group

    a. Interferon ß-1b (Betaseron) 250 micrograms subcutaneously every other day

    b. Placebo injected subcutaneously every other day

3. Results: diagnosis of CDMS established or follow-up of 2 years

    a. Reduction of development of CDMS over 2 years from 45% (placebo) to 28% (treatment)

    b. Similar significant reduction at 2 years if McDonald criteria (combines clinical and MRI findings) used: 51% (placebo) vs 28% (treatment)

Table 9-3

AMERICAN COLLEGE OF RHEUMATOLOGY CRITERIA FOR CLASSIFICATION OF GIANT CELL ARTERITIS

1. Age at onset of 50 years or older
2. Onset of new headache
3. Temporal artery abnormality (tender or reduced pulsation)
4. Elevated ESR defined as >50 mm/hour using Westergren method
5. Abnormal artery biopsy showing necrotizing vasculitis with predominant mononuclear cell infiltration or granulomatous inflammation

Sensitivity 93.5%, specificity 91.2% for diagnosis with at least three of five criteria met.

        c.   At the 25th percentile, time to develop CDMS was delayed from 255 days (placebo) to 618 days (treatment)

  Q.   Results of CHAMPS, ETOMS, and BENEFIT all strongly support use of interferon therapy in patients presenting with a first clinical event suggestive of multiple sclerosis

VI. Ischemic optic neuropathy (ION)

  A.   Ischemic infarction of the anterior portion of the optic nerve

  B.   Acute visual loss, usually in patients over the age of 60

  C.   Clinical settings in which ION is seen
     1.   Arterial disease
        a.   Arteritis
            i.   Giant cell arteritis (Table 9-3)
            ii.   Collagen vascular diseases
           iii.   Syphilis
           iv.   Herpes zoster
        b.   Nonarteritic ischemic optic neuropathy (NAION)—"arteriosclerosis"
        c.   Diabetes mellitus
        d.   Malignant hypertension
        e.   Embolic disease
        f.   Vasospastic (migraine)
        g.   Post-irradiation
     2.   Hypotension/hypovolemia
        a.   Massive blood loss
        b.   Cardiac insufficiency
        c.   Surgical hypotension
        d.   Anemia
     3.   Other
        a.   Post-cataract surgery
        b.   Amiodarone

  D.   Differential diagnosis involves arteritic (giant cell arteritis) vs nonarteritic (arteriosclerotic) as major causes of ION (Table 9-4)

	Table 9-4	

MAJOR CAUSES OF ISCHEMIC OPTIC NEUROPATHY

	NAION	**Giant Cell Arteritis**
Age peak	60 to 70 years	70 to 80 years
Visual loss	Minimal to severe	Usually severe
Involvement of second eye	Approximately 40%	Approximately 75%
Acute fundus	Swollen disc	Swollen disc, may be pallid
Other ophthalmologic presentations		Central retinal artery occlusion, choroidal infarction, anterior segment ischemia
Systemic	Hypertension (approximately 50%)	Headache, scalp tenderness, malaise, weakness, weight loss, fever, jaw pain, polymyalgia
ESR (Westergren, mm/hour)	Up to 40	Usually high (50 to 120)
CRP (C reactive protein, mg/dL)*	Normal	Elevated
Temporal artery biopsy	May show arteriosclerotic change	Granulomatous inflammation, multinucleated giant cells, disruption of internal elastic lamina
Response to steroids	None	Relief of systemic symptoms, infrequent return of vision, protect other eye

*Normal range established by individual laboratory.
Modified from Glaser JS. *Neuro-Ophthalmology*. 3rd ed. Philadelphia, Pa: Lippincott Williams & Wilkins; 1999:163.

E. ION is virtually always accompanied by disc swelling in the acute stage; rare exception in posterior ION associated with giant cell arteritis

F. Optic disc in NAION is commonly full and cupless ("disc at risk")

G. Visual defect is usually maximal in onset. On occasion, field abnormality may progress within the first month. Subsequent improvement may occur in up to 40% of patients with NAION

H. With arteritic ION, may see marked delay in choroidal perfusion with fluorescein angiography: signifies involvement of posterior ciliary arteries

I. Recognition of cases due to giant cell arteritis is essential; prompt steroid therapy may restore some degree of vision, avert visual loss in the fellow eye, and improve long-term systemic morbidity and mortality

VII. Miscellaneous causes of swollen optic disc

A. Orbital disease

1. Optic nerve or arachnoid cyst

2. Orbital tumor

3. Dysthyroid optic neuropathy (see Chapter 11, V)

        a.   Unilateral or bilateral progressive visual loss

        b.   Patient may have only mild to moderate congestive, orbital signs

        c.   Visual field loss typically central scotoma, sometimes combined with inferior depression

        d.   Optic disc may appear swollen, normal, or pale

        e.   Optic neuropathy due to compression of optic nerve by enlarged extra-ocular muscles at orbital apex

        f.   Treatment: systemic steroids, radiotherapy, orbital decompression surgery

B. Intraocular disease: uveitis, vein occlusion, disc tumor, hypotony

C. Diabetic papillopathy (diabetic papillitis, "acute disc swelling in juvenile diabetes")

    1.   Onset: second to eighth decades (average: 50 years)

    2.   Type I or II diabetics of some chronicity (average: 10 to 12 years)

    3.   Commonly bilateral but may be unilateral

    4.   Disc edema with prominent telangiectatic change without neovascularization

    5.   No correlation with degree of diabetic retinopathy

    6.   Frequently asymptomatic or modest acuity loss to 20/50; occasionally more profound loss

    7.   Visual field defects include enlarged blind spot and arcuate defects

    8.   Generally good visual prognosis with return of normal acuity in 3 months to 1 year

    9.   Visual improvement precedes disappearance of disc swelling

    10.   Disc usually regains normal appearance, although may also develop diffuse or segmental pallor

D. Papillophlebitis (retinal vasculitis, optic disc vasculitis, big blind spot syndrome)

    1.   Usually unilateral disc edema

    2.   Young, healthy adults

    3.   Vague visual complaints of blurred vision with minimal impairment of acuity (usually no worse than 20/30)

    4.   No afferent pupillary defect

    5.   Only visual field abnormality is enlargement of blind spot

    6.   Disc swelling with associated engorged retinal veins and occasional retinal hemorrhages

    7.   Spontaneous, usually complete recovery within several months to 1 year

    8.   Pathologic examination reveals inflammation of the retinal veins, although etiology of inflammation is unknown

E. Leber's hereditary optic neuropathy (see Table 10-1)

    1.   Most often, but not exclusively, affects males in the second or third decade of life

    2.   Rapid monocular visual loss to a variable level (20/200 or worse)

    3.   Second eye usually affected within days or weeks

    4.   In acute phase, optic disc may appear normal or have typical triad of findings

        a.   Circumpapillary telangiectatic microangiopathy

         b.   Prominent NFL around disc

         c.   Absence of dye leakage from the disc or peripapillary region with fluorescein angiography

   5.   Visual field abnormality is centrocecal scotoma

   6.   Ultimately, the patient develops either temporal or generalized disc pallor

   7.   Maternal inheritance pattern in Leber's hereditary optic neuropathy

         a.   Disorder of mitochondrial, not chromosomal, DNA

         b.   Chromosomal DNA follows Mendelian pattern of inheritance, but mitochondrial DNA is inherited exclusively from the mother

         c.   Leber's optic neuropathy linked with several point mutations in mitochondrial DNA, most commonly 11778, but also 14484, 3460

         d.   Mitochondrial DNA is essential for oxydative phosphorylation, the energy-producing cycle in the cell

         e.   Heteroplasmy: intracellular mitochondrial DNA is a mixture of mutant and normal forms; provides basis for variable clinical expression of mutation

   8.   Electrocardiogram obtained to exclude potential cardiac conduction defect

   9.   No effective treatment—eliminate use of tobacco, alcohol

   10.   Rarely, spontaneous recovery of vision may occur (frequency based on genetic mutation: 14484 > 3460 > 11778)

F.   Spheno-orbital meningioma

   1.   Chronic compression of the intraorbital or intracanalicular optic nerve (see Chapter 10, VI, B)

   2.   Clinical triad

         a.   Visual loss

         b.   Optic disc swelling that resolves into optic atrophy

         c.   Appearance of optociliary shunt vessels

   3.   The clinical picture may also be seen with optic nerve glioma, chronic papilledema, craniopharyngioma

G.   Optic disc edema with macular star

   1.   Descriptive term that includes several different disease processes

   2.   Main clinical settings:

         a.   Inflammatory papillitis

         b.   Vascular disorders (hypertension, diabetes mellitus)

         c.   Papilledema

         d.   Infectious/immune mediated

   3.   Neuroretinitis is a general description often applied to infectious/immune-mediated cause

   4.   Leber's idiopathic stellate neuroretinitis

         a.   Triad: visual loss, optic disc edema, macular star

         b.   Children and young adults

         c.   Antecedent viral illness in up to 50% of patients

         d.   Generally benign, self-limited condition

         e.   Resolution of disc edema in 3 months; up to 1 year for macular star to resolve

      f.   Visual prognosis usually good
5.   Neuroretinitis may be due to organisms other than virus:
      a.   Cat scratch disease (Bartonella henselae)
      b.   Toxoplasmosis
      c.   Toxocariasis
      d.   Histoplasmosis
      e.   Spirochetoses (syphilis, Lyme disease)

H.   Paraneoplastic optic neuropathy
1.   Subacute, progressive, usually bilateral visual loss without pain
2.   Optic disc usually edematous; may be normal
3.   Usually part of paraneoplastic brainstem or cerebellar syndrome
4.   Reported with variety of cancers, including:
      a.   Small-cell lung carcinoma
      b.   Hodgkin's and non-Hodgkin's lymphoma
      c.   Neuroblastoma
      d.   Neuropharyngeal cancer
      e.   Thymoma
5.   Must rule out direct compression or infiltration of the optic nerve
6.   Check serum for collapsin response-mediated protein-5 (CRMP-5) antibodies: IgG antibodies directed against antigen expressed in neural tissues and associated neoplasms
7.   Pathology: perivascular inflammation, axonal loss, demyelination
8.   Significant visual improvement may occur following chemotherapy and/or radiation therapy

VIII. Pseudopapilledema (anomalous elevation of the disc; congenitally full disc)

A.   Ophthalmoscopic features
1.   Disc is not hyperemic, and there are no dilated capillaries on its surface
2.   Despite disc elevation, surface arteries are not obscured (no peripapillary NFL opacification)
3.   Physiologic cup usually absent
4.   May see anomalous branching and tortuosity of retinal vessels (abnormally large number of branches at disc margin)
5.   May see drusen (hyaline bodies) buried in disc of patient or relatives
6.   No hemorrhages (rare exceptions)
7.   No exudates or cotton-wool spots
8.   Disc usually has irregular border with pigment epithelial defects in peripapillary retina
9.   Visual field testing may show enlarged blind spots and nerve fiber bundle defects

B.   If exam is suggestive of buried disc drusen, may use orbital ultrasonography or CT to "visualize" them

BIBLIOGRAPHY

Books

Digre KB, Corbett JJ. *Practical Viewing of the Optic Disc*. Boston, Mass: Butterworth-Heinemann; 2003.

Kline LB, Foroozan R, eds. Optic nerve disorders. *Ophthalmology Monographs*. Vol 10. San Francisco, Calif: American Academy of Ophthalmology; 2007.

Chapters

Glaser JS. *Neuro-Ophthalmology*. 3rd ed. Philadelphia, Pa: Lippincott Williams & Wilkins; 1999:118-197.

Martin TJ, Corbett JJ. *Neuro-Ophthalmology—The Requisites*. St Louis, Mo: Mosby; 2000:57-94.

Articles

Appen RE, de Venecia G, Ferwerda J. Optic disc vasculitis. *Am J Ophthalmol*. 1980;90:352-359.

Barr CC, Glaser JS, Blankenship G. Acute disc swelling in juvenile diabetes. Clinical profile and natural history of 12 cases. *Arch Ophthalmol*. 1980;92:2185-2192.

Brodsky MC, Vaphiades M. Magnetic resonance imaging in pseudotumor cerebri. *Ophthalmology*. 1998;105:1686-1693.

Chan JW. Paraneoplastic retinopathies and optic neuropathies. *Surv Ophthalmol*. 2003;48:12-38.

Cogan DG. Blackouts not obviously due to carotid occlusion. *Arch Ophthalmol*. 1961;66:180-187.

Comi G, Fillipi M, Barkhof F, et al. Effect of early interferon treatment on conversion to definite multiple sclerosis: a randomized study. *Lancet*. 2001;357:1576-1582.

Cross SA, Salamao DR, Parisi JE, et al. Paraneoplastic autoimmune optic neuritis with retinitis defined by CRMP-5-IgG. *Ann Neurol*. 2003;54:38-50.

Flippi M, Rovaris M, Ingles M, et al. Interferon beta-1a for brain tissue loss in patients at presentation with syndrome suggestive of multiple sclerosis: a randomized, double-blind, placebo-controlled trial. *Lancet*. 2004;364:1489-1496.

Friedman DI, Jacobson DM. Idiopathic intracranial hypertension. *J Neuroophthalmol*. 2004;24:138-145.

Frisén L, Hoyt WF, Tengroth BM. Optociliary veins, disc pallor, and visual loss: a triad of signs indicating spheno-orbital meningioma. *Acta Ophthalmol*. 1973;51:241-249.

Ischemic Optic Neuropathy Decompression Trial Research Group. Optic nerve decompression surgery for nonarteritic ischemic optic neuropathy is not effective and may be harmful. *JAMA*. 1995;273:625-632.

Jacobs LD, Beck RW, Simon JH, et al. Intramuscular interferon beta 1-a therapy initiated during a first demyelinating event in multiple sclerosis. CHAMPS study group. *N Engl J Med*. 2000;343:898-904.

Johnson LN, Krohel GB, Madsen RW, March GA. The role of weight loss and acetazolamide in the treatment of idiopathic intracranial hypertension (pseudotumor cerebri). *Ophthalmology*. 1998;105:2313-2317.

Kappos L, Polman CH, Freedman MS. Treatment with interferon beta-1b delays conversion to clinically definite and McDonald MS in patient with clinically isolated syndromes. *Neurology*. 2006;67:1-8.

Kesler A, Bassan H. Pseudotumor cerebri–idiopathic intracranial hypertension in the pediatric population. *Pediatric Endocrinology Reviews*. 2006;4:387-392.

Lennon VA, Wingerchuk DM, Kryzen TJ, et al. A serum autoantibody marker of neuromyelitis optica: distinction from multiple sclerosis. *Lancet*. 2004;364:2106-2112.

Levin BE. The clinical significance of spontaneous pulsations of the retinal vein. *Arch Neurol*. 1978;35:37-40.

Lonn LI, Hoyt WF. Papillophlebitis: a cause of protracted yet benign optic disc edema. *Eye Ear Nose Throat Monthly*. 1966;45:62-68.

Miller GR, Smith JL. Ischemic optic neuropathy. *Am J Ophthalmol*. 1966;62:103-115.

Minkler DS, Tso MOM, Zimmerman LE. A light microscopic, autoradiographic study of axoplasmic transport in the optic nerve head during ocular hypotony, increased intracranial pressure, and papilledema. *Am J Ophthalmol*. 1976;82:741-759.

Monheit BE, Read RW. Optic disc edema associated with sudden-onset anterior uveitis. *Am J Ophthalmol*. 2005;140:733-735.

Morgan JE. Circulation and axonal transport in the optic nerve. *Eye*. 2004;18:1089-1095.

Okun E. Chronic papilledema simulating hyaline bodies of the optic disc. *Am J Ophthalmol*. 1962;53:922-927.

Optic Neuritis Study Group. High- and low-risk profiles for the development of multiple sclerosis within 10 years after optic neuritis. *Arch Ophthalmol*. 2003;121:944-949.

Regillo CP, Brown GC, Savino PJ, et al. Diabetic papillopathy. *Arch Ophthalmol*. 1995;113:889-895.

Smith JL, Hoyt WF, Susac JO. Ocular fundus in acute Leber's optic neuropathy. *Arch Ophthalmol*. 1973;90:349-354.

Solley A, Martin DF, Newman NJ. Cat scratch disease. Posterior segment manifestation. *Ophthalmology*. 1999;106:1546-1553.

Spencer WH. Drusen of the optic disc and aberrant axoplasmic transport. The XXIII Edward Jackson Memorial Lecture. *Am J Ophthalmol*. 1978;85:1-12.

Thuente DD, Buckley EG. Pediatric optic nerve sheath decompression. *Ophthalmology*. 2005;112:724-727.

Tso MO, Hayreh SS. Optic disc edema in raised intracranial pressure: III. A pathologic study of experimental papilledema. *Arch Ophthalmol*. 1977;95:1448-1457.

Tso MO, Hayreh SS. Optic disc edema in raised intracranial pressure: IV. Axoplasmic transport in experimental papilledema. *Arch Ophthalmol*. 1977;95:1458-1462.

Wingerchuk DM, Hogancamp WF, O'Brien PC, Weinshenker BG. The clinical course of neuromyelitis optica (Devic's syndrome). *Neurology*. 1999;53:1107-1114.

Chapter 10

The Pale Optic Disc: Optic Atrophy

Lanning B. Kline, MD

I. **Optic disc pallor vs optic atrophy**

   A. Ophthalmoscopic appearance of disc pallor alone does not establish the presence of optic atrophy

   B. Frequently, the temporal side of the normal disc has less color than the nasal side

   C. Optic atrophy is a pathologic description of optic nerve shrinkage from any process that produces degeneration of axons in the anterior visual system (retinogeniculate) pathway

   D. The clinical diagnosis of optic atrophy is based on:
   1. Ophthalmoscopic abnormalities of color and structure of the disc with associated changes in retinal vessels and nerve fiber layer (NFL)
   2. Defective visual function (acuity, color vision pupils, fields, visual evoked response) and can be localized to the optic nerve

II. **Histopathologic considerations**

   A. When a visual axon is severed, its ascending (to the brain) segment disintegrates and disappears in approximately 7 days. This is termed wallerian degeneration

   B. The portion of the axon still connected to the ganglion cell body remains viable for 3 to 4 weeks but then rapidly degenerates by 6 to 8 weeks. This is called descending (to the eye) degeneration

   C. With the completion of descending degeneration of axons, optic disc pallor appears. Currently, there are two major theories to explain acquired disc pallor
   1. Vascular-glial theory: when the optic nerve degenerates, its blood supply is reduced and smaller vessels, recognizable in the normal disc, disappear from view. In addition, formation of glial tissue at the nerve head is said to occur with optic atrophy
   2. NFL theory (Figure 10-1): with degeneration of visual axons, there is alteration in the thickness and cytoarchitecture of nerve fiber bundles passing between glial columns containing capillaries. Alteration of light conducted along the nerve fiber bundles leads to the appearance of pallor, and there is no reduction in blood supply to the optic disc

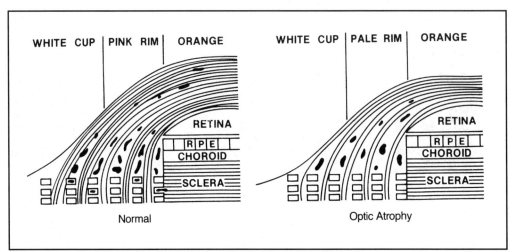

Figure 10-1. Schematic drawing of the longitudinal section of normal and atrophic optic discs. In optic atrophy, there is a decrease in the number of nerve fibers and capillaries, but the proportion of capillaries per unit volume is unchanged. (Modified from Quigley HA, Anderson DR. The histologic basis of optic disc pallor in experimental optic atrophy. *Am J Ophthalmol.* 1977;83:709-717.)

III.   Ophthalmoscopic features of optic atrophy

A.   As a general rule, fundus signs are not specific for any particular etiology of optic atrophy, and the diagnosis must be obtained from nonophthalmoscopic findings

B.   In the early stages of atrophy, the optic disc loses its reddish hue, and the substance of the disc slowly melts away to leave a pale, shallow concave meniscus—the exposed lamina cribrosa

C.   Ipsilateral attenuation of the retinal arterioles is frequently a sign of old central retinal artery occlusion

D.   Healed papillitis or ischemic optic neuropathy may cause narrowing of retinal arterioles only in their peripapillary segment, after which they appear to enlarge slightly in caliber as they traverse the fundus ("reverse taper sign")

E.   Pathologic disc cupping may develop, along with disc pallor, in patients without glaucoma. Etiologies include ischemia, compression, inflammation, and trauma. Findings that indicated optic disc excavation is nonglaucomatous include:

1.   Decreased visual acuity out of proportion to amount of cupping or visual field loss

2.   Acquired dyschromatopsia

3.   Visual field defects out of proportion to degree of cupping

4.   Visual field defects not typical of glaucoma (central scotoma; defects align along vertical meridian)

5.   Optic disc pallor out of proportion to the degree of cupping

F.   During fundus examination, NFL defects should be carefully looked for when suspecting optic atrophy. They appear as dark slits or wedges and are most easily identified in the superior and inferior arcuate regions where the NFL is particularly thick. Also, vessels in this area, having lost their surrounding nerve fiber covering, appear darker than normal and stand out sharply

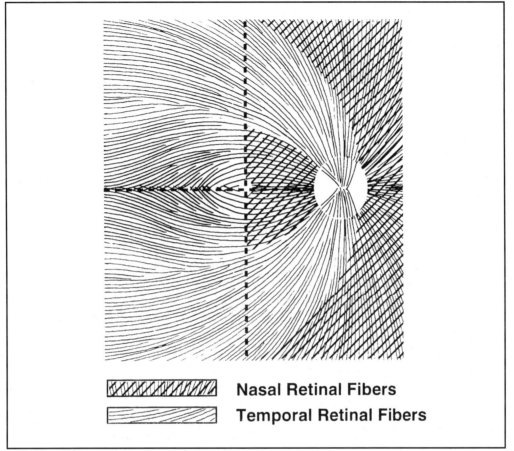

Nasal Retinal Fibers

Temporal Retinal Fibers

Figure 10-2. Bow-tie atrophy. With long-standing chiasmal compression, the nasal retinal fibers become atrophic, and pallor is seen in a pattern corresponding to the location of the fibers in the optic disc. (Modified from Newman NJ. Chiasm, parachiasmal syndromes, retrochiasm and disorders of higher visual function. In: Slamovits TL, Burde RM, eds. *Neuro-Ophthalmology*. St Louis, Mo: Mosby-Year Book; 1994:4-7.)

    G.   "Bow-tie" or "band" optic atrophy (Figure 10-2)

        1.   Specific patterns of NFL and optic atrophy from optic chiasmal and retrochiasmal-pregeniculate lesions

        2.   With temporal field defects, loss of nerve fiber from ganglion cells nasal to fovea

        3.   Results in atrophy of nasal and temporal portions of the disc, with relative sparing of superior and inferior arcuate bundles

        4.   Arcuate bundles are spared since they arise from ganglion cells both temporal and nasal to the fovea

    H.   Optic nerve hypoplasia

        1.   Incomplete development of the optic nerve

        2.   Unilateral or bilateral

        3.   Variable acuity depending upon degree of development

        4.   Double ring sign: hypoplastic disc surrounded by ring of sclera and ring of hyperpigmentation

        5.   Clinical settings:

            a.   Unilateral: isolated or accompanied by strabismus and/or nystagmus

            b.   Bilateral: forebrain malformation and endocrinologic defects

                i.   Septo-optic dysplasia (de Morsier's syndrome)

                ii.   Short stature

                iii.   Absence of septum pellucidum, corpus callosum

                iv.   Endocrine deficits: growth hormone, hypothyroidism, sexual development, diabetes insipidus

                v.   Association with cortical migration disorders: schizencephaly, pachygyria, cortical heterotopias

        6.   Associated conditions

            a.   Maternal diabetes mellitus

            b.   Fetal alcohol syndrome

            c.   Use during pregnancy of LSD, quinine, antiepileptic drugs

        7.   Patient evaluation (bilateral cases)

            a.   Cranial magnetic resonance imaging (MRI): with endocrine abnormalities often find posterior pituitary ectopia or absence of posterior pituitary infundibulum

            b.   Endocrinologic and neurologic evaluations

I.   Homonymous hemioptic hypoplasia

        1.   Optic disc findings in patients with congenital cerebral hemiatrophy, presumably due to fetal vascular insufficiency

        2.   Fundus ipsilateral to hemispheric defect shows slightly small optic disc with temporal pallor and loss of NFL of ganglion cells temporal to the fovea

        3.   Fundus contralateral to hemispheric defect shows small disc with "band" atrophy

        4.   Associated findings include mental retardation, seizures, congenital hemiplegia, and complete homonymous hemianopia

J.   Superior segmental optic hypoplasia

        1.   Ophthalmoscopic findings

            a.   Bilateral

            b.   Superior entrance of central retinal artery into optic disc

            c.   Pallor of superior disc

            d.   Superior peripapillary halo

            e.   Thinning of superior NFL

        2.   Inferior visual field deficits of which patient may be unaware

        3.   Often found in children of diabetic mothers

K.   Morning Glory disc anomaly

        1.   Ophthalmoscopic findings

            a.   Unilateral

            b.   Enlarged, funnel-shaped, excavated optic disc

            c.   Surrounded by annulus of chorioretinal pigmentary disturbance

      2.   Vision usually poor

      3.   May lead to retinal detachment

      4.   Occurrence:

           a.   Isolated

           b.   Basal encephalocele

           c.   Pituitary dwarfism

           d.   Moyamoya disease

           e.   Neurofibromatosis—type 2

  L.   Papillorenal (renal-coloboma) syndrome

      1.   Triad of:

           a.   Optic disc "coloboma"—multiple cilioretinal vessels

           b.   Renal hypoplasia/insufficiency

           c.   PAX 2 genetic mutation

      2.   Additional clinical features

           a.   May develop retinal detachment

           b.   Central nervous system (CNS) abnormalities: microcephaly, mental retardation

           c.   Auditory: high-frequency hearing loss

IV. Hereditary optic neuropathies

  A.   These forms of optic nerve disease often cause insidious, bilateral, symmetric loss of central acuity (see Chapter 9, VII, E)

  B.   Table 10-1 summarizes the major forms of hereditary optic nerve disease

V. Toxic and deficiency optic neuropathies

  A.   Particular forms of medical therapy or exposure to specific toxins may lead to bilateral retrobulbar optic neuropathy, characterized by visual loss, severe dyschromatopsia, central field defects with occasional peripheral field constriction, and initially normal-appearing optic discs that may gradually become pale

  B.   Medication-induced toxic optic neuropathies

      1.   Antibiotics

           a.   Ethambutol

           b.   Isoniazid

           c.   Streptomycin

           d.   Rifampin

           e.   Halogenated hydroquinolones

           f.   Linezolid

      2.   Immunosuppressants/immunomodulators

           a.   Cyclosporine

           b.   Tacrolimus

           c.   Interferon

      3.   Chemotherapeutic agents

           a.   Cisplatinum

           b.   Carboplatinum

           c.   Nitrosoureas: BCNU, CCNU

           d.   Vincristine

Table 10-1

HEREDOFAMILIAL OPTIC ATROPHIES

| | Disorders of Chromosomal DNA | | | | Disorders of Mitochondrial DNA |
| | Dominant | | Recessive | | Maternal |
	Juvenile (infantile)	Early infantile (congenital); simple	Behr's type; complicated	With diabetes mellitus ± deafness	Leber's disease
Age at onset	Childhood (4 to 8 years)	Early childhood* (3 to 4 years)	Childhood (1 to 9 years)	Childhood (6 to 14 years)	Early adulthood (18 to 30 years, up to sixth decade)
Visual impairment	Mild/moderate (20/40 to 20/200)	Severe (20/200 to HM)	Moderate (20/200)	Severe (20/400 to FC)	Moderate/severe (20/200 to FC)
Nystagmus	Rare**	Usual	In 50%	Absent	Absent
Optic disc	Mild temporal pallor ± temporal excavation†	Marked diffuse pallor ± arteriolar attenuation†	Mild temporal pallor	Marked diffuse pallor	Moderate diffuse pallor; Disc swelling in acute phase
Color vision	Blue-yellow dyschromatopsia	Severe dyschromatopsia/achromatopsia	Moderate to severe dyschromatopsia	Severe dyschromatopsia	Dense central scotoma for colors
Course	Variable, slight progression	Stable	Stable	Progressive	Acute visual loss, then usually stable, may improve/worsen

FC=finger counting, HM=hand motions.

*Difficult to assess in infancy, but visual impairment usually manifests by age 4 years.

**Presence of nystagmus with poor vision and earlier onset suggests separate congenital or infantile form.

†Distinguished from tapetoretinal degenerations by normal electroretinogram (ERG).

Modified from Glaser JS. Neuro-Ophthalmology. 3rd ed. Philadelphia, Pa: Lippincott Williams & Wilkins; 1999:128.

      4.   Cardiac medications

         a.   Digitalis

         b.   Amiodarone

      5.   Miscellaneous

         a.   Disulfiram

         b.   Chlorpropamide

  C.   Grant's *Toxicology of the Eye* lists over 20 toxins associated with optic neuropathy including:

      1.   Arsenic

      2.   Lead

      3.   Hexachlorophene (Phisohex [Sanofi-Aventis, Bridgewater, NJ])

      4.   Methanol

      5.   Lysol

      6.   Quinine

      7.   Ethylene glycol

      8.   Toluene

  D.   Deficiency optic neuropathies

      1.   Clinical picture of progressive bilateral visual loss, with central or centrocecal scotomas and some degree of temporal disc pallor and atrophy of the papillomacular NFL

      2.   Vitamin deficiencies that may be responsible for optic atrophy include:

         a   Vitamin B_{12} (cobalamin)

         b.   Vitamin B_6 (pyridoxine)

         c.   Vitamin B_1 (thiamine)

         d.   Niacin

         e.   Vitamin B_2 (riboflavin)

         f.   Folic acid

  E.   Tobacco-alcohol amblyopia

      1.   Similar clinical picture to deficiency optic neuropathies listed above

      2.   Continuing controversy as to whether this represents a form of toxic (cyanide) or deficiency (vitamin) optic nerve disease

      3.   In general, prognosis for recovery of vision is good except in the most chronic cases

VI. Primary optic nerve neoplasms

  A.   Optic glioma

      1.   Two major forms: childhood (benign) and adulthood (malignant) (Table 10-2)

      2.   Childhood form

         a.   Patient presents with visual loss, proptosis, occasionally monocular nystagmus ("spasmus nutans," see Chapter 3)

         b.   One/both optic nerves and/or chiasm

         c.   Up to 25% may have neurofibromatosis (see Chapter 19, II)

         d.   Neuroimaging: double-intensity tubular thickening and kinking of orbital optic nerve(s), enlargement of chiasm, infiltration of hypothalamus

Table 10-2

PRIMARY GLIOMAS OF THE OPTIC NERVE AND CHIASM

	Childhood	Adulthood
Age at onset of symptoms	4 to 8 years	Middle age
Presentation	Visual loss, proptosis	Rapid severe visual loss
Course	Relatively stable, nonprogressive	Rapid bilateral visual deterioration, other intracranial signs (eg, confusion, lethargy)
Prognosis	Compatible with long life	Death within months to 2 years
Neurofibromatosis	Associated in up to 25% of cases	No relationship
Histology	Pilocytic astrocytoma	Malignant astrocytoma (glioblastoma); may metastasize

Modified from Glaser JS. *Neuro-Ophthalmology*. 3rd ed. Philadelphia, Pa: Lippincott Williams & Wilkins; 1999:218.

    e.   Visual pathway gliomas may remain stable, enlarge, or regress (post-biopsy or spontaneously)

    f.   Treatment controversial: observation, surgery, radiation therapy, chemotherapy

  3. Adult form

    a.   Rapid onset of visual loss and relentless deterioration

    b.   Usually begins in chiasm

    c.   Neuroimaging: suprasellar mass with edema

    d.   Treatment: radiation only palliative

B.   Optic nerve sheath meningioma

  1. Typically occurs in young to middle-aged women

  2. Insidious, progressive visual loss

  3. Most commonly unilateral, but may be bilateral

  4. May be associated with neurofibromatosis type 2

  5. Optic disc chronically swollen, becomes pale, with appearance of optociliary shunt vessels

  6. Neuroimaging

    a.   Computed tomography (CT): "tram-track" appearance due to calcification

    b.   MRI: enhancement with intravenous gadolinium; able to detect intracranial spread through optic canal

  7. Treatment: radiation therapy; surgery with evidence of intracranial progression

VII. Infiltrative optic neuropathy

A.   Optic disc initially swollen or normal; ultimately becomes pale

B.   Often acute visual loss

C. Etiology may be benign or malignant
  1. Sarcoidosis
  2. Lymphoma
  3. Leukemia
  4. Plasmacytoma
  5. Malignant histiocytosis

VIII. Carcinomatous optic neuropathy

  A. Fundus typically normal at onset of visual loss, with disc gradually becoming pale

  B. Patient may or may not have history of known malignancy

  C. Optic neuropathy may be isolated or accompanied by other neurologic defects

  D. Visual loss typically acute and devastating

  E. Unless large intraparenchymal CNS spread has occurred, radiologic studies (CT, MRI, angiography) are often normal

  F. May see meningeal enhancement with cranial MR scanning following IV contrast

  G. Careful cerebrospinal fluid analysis with cytologic examination for malignant cells

  H. Due to microscopic infiltrates of the nerve and its sheaths

IX. Radiation optic neuropathy

  A. Due to delayed radionecrosis of optic nerve and chiasm

  B. Follows radiation therapy (external beam, gamma knife) for perisellar tumor, such as pituitary adenoma, craniopharyngioma, invasive sinus carcinoma

  C. Diagnostic criteria
  1. Acute visual loss (monocular or binocular)
  2. Visual field defects indicating optic nerve or chiasmal dysfunction
  3. Optic disc edema usually absent (see Chapter 9, VI)
  4. Onset usually within 3 years of therapy (peak: 1 to 1.5 years)
  5. Neuroimaging studies demonstrate no evidence of anterior visual pathway compression
  6. Contrast-enhanced MR scanning may demonstrate areas of increased signal in optic nerves and/or chiasm

  D. Pathology: fibrinoid necrosis of blood vessels, demyelination, necrosis

  E. Treatment: none of proven efficacy

X. Traumatic optic neuropathy

  A. Three categories:
  1. Evulsion
  2. Direct injury
  3. Indirect injury

  B. Optic nerve evulsion
  1. Dislocation of optic nerve from scleral canal
  2. Partial or complete
  3. As early vitreous hemorrhage clears optic disc partially or totally absent
  4. May be confirmed with imaging studies (ultrasound, CT, MRI)
  5. Treatment: none

C.   Direct injury
1.   Impact on optic nerve or its sheaths by a blunt or sharp object
2.   With anterior injury, may see fundus picture of central retinal artery occlusion (CRAO)
3.   More posterior involvement leads to normal fundus appearance followed by optic atrophy within 4 to 8 weeks
4.   Multiple pathophysiologic mechanisms
    a.   Laceration
    b.   Bone deformation/fracture
    c.   Vascular insufficiency
    d.   Hemorrhage
5.   Imaging studies: CT, MRI (contraindicated with ferromagnetic foreign body)
6.   Treatment individualized; megadose intravenous steroids, surgery

D.   Indirect injury
1.   Blunt trauma to orbit or cranium with lines of force transmitted to orbital apex
2.   Most common form of traumatic optic neuropathy
3.   Canalicular optic nerve is site of injury
4.   Fundus initially normal with appearance of optic atrophy in 4 to 8 weeks
5.   Imaging studies may be normal or demonstrate optic canal fracture
6.   Pathophysiologic mechanisms, as with direct injury (see above)
7.   Treatment: none of proven efficacy

BIBLIOGRAPHY

Books

Digre KB, Corbett JJ. *Practical Viewing of the Optic Disc.* Boston, Mass: Butterworth-Heinemann; 2003.

Grant M, Schuman JS. *Toxicology of the Eye.* 4th ed. Springfield, Ill: Thomas; 1993.

Kline LB, Foroozan R, eds. Optic nerve disorders. *Ophthalmology Monographs.* Vol 10. San Francisco, Calif: American Academy of Ophthalmology; 2007.

Articles

Andrews DW, Foroozan R, Yang BP, et al. Fractionated stereotactic radiotherapy for the treatment of optic nerve sheath meningiomas. *Neurosurgery.* 2002;51:890-904.

Carrasco JR, Penne RB. Optic nerve sheath meningiomas and advanced treatment options. *Curr Opin Ophthalmol.* 2004;15:406-410.

Hoyt WF, Rios-Montenegro EN, Behrens MM, et al. Homonymous hemioptic hypoplasia: funduscopic features in standard and red-free illumination in three patients with congenital hemiplegia. *Br J Ophthalmol.* 1972;56:537-545.

Imes RK, Hoyt WF. Childhood chiasmal gliomas: update on the fate of patients in the 1969 San Francisco study. *Br J Ophthalmol.* 1986;70:179-182.

Jacobson DM. Gliomas of the anterior visual pathways. *Neurosurg Clin N Am.* 1999;10:683-698.

Kline LB, Kim JY, Ceballos R. Radiation optic neuropathy. *Ophthalmology.* 1985,92:1118-1126.

Levin LA, Beck RW, Joseph JP. The treatment of traumatic optic neuropathy: the international optic nerve trauma study. *Ophthalmology.* 1999;106:1268-1277.

Liu GT. Optic gliomas of the anterior visual pathway. *Curr Opin Ophthalmol.* 2006;17:427-431.

Newman NJ. Hereditary optic neuropathies: from the mitochondria to the optic nerve. *Am J Ophthalmol.* 2005;140:517-523.

Parsa C, Hoyt CS, Lesser RL, et al. Spontaneous regression of optic nerve glioma: thirteen cases documented by serial neuroimaging. *Arch Ophthalmol.* 2001;119:516-529.

Parsa CF, Silva ED, Sundin OH, et al. Redefining papillorenal syndrome: an underdiagnosed cause of ocular and renal morbidity. *Ophthalmology.* 2001;108:733-749.

Rucker JC, Hamilton SR, Bardenstein D, et al. Linezolid-associated toxic optic neuropathy. *Neurology.* 2006;66:595-598.

Saeed P, Rootman J, Nugent RA, et al. Optic nerve sheath meningioma. *Ophthalmology.* 2003;110:2019-2030.

Siatkowski RM, Sanchez JC, Androde R, et al. The clinical, neuroradiographic, and endocrinologic profile of patients with bilateral optic nerve hypoplasia. *Ophthalmology.* 1197;104:493-496.

Steinsapir KD, Goldberg RA. Traumatic optic neuropathy. *Surv Ophthalmol.* 1994;38:487-518.

Trobe JD, Glaser JS, Cassady JC, et al. Nonglaucomatous excavation of the optic disc. *Arch Ophthalmol.* 1980;98:1046-1050.

Turbin RE, Thompson CR, Kennerdell JS, et al. A long-term visual outcome comparison in patients with optic nerve sheath meningioma managed with observation, surgery, radiotherapy, or surgery and radiotherapy. *Ophthalmology.* 2002;109:890-900.

Unsöld R, Hoyt WF. Band atrophy of the optic nerve. The histology of temporal hemianopsia. *Arch Ophthalmol.* 1980;98:1637-1638.

Victor M. Tobacco alcohol amblyopia: a critique of current concepts of this disorder, with special reference to the role of nutritional deficiency in its causation. *Arch Ophthalmol.* 1963;70:313-318.

Yen MY, Wang AG, Wei YH. Leber's hereditary optic neuropathy: a multifunctional disease. *Prog Retin Eye Res.* 2006;25:381-395.

Chapter 11

Myasthenia and Ocular Myopathies

Lanning B. Kline, MD

I. **Myasthenia and ocular myopathies**

    A.   These disorders produce ocular motor dysfunction due to involvement of the extraocular muscles and the neuromuscular junction

    B.   Some of these entities may simulate isolated or combined ocular motor cranial nerve palsies

II. **Myasthenia gravis**

    A.   Disease characterized clinically by muscle weakness and fatigue

    B.   It is the most common disorder affecting the neuromuscular junction

    C.   Myasthenia involves skeletal and not visceral musculature; therefore, the pupil and ciliary muscle are unaffected. Major ophthalmologic complaints are ptosis and diplopia

    D.   Ocular involvement eventually occurs in 90% of myasthenics and accounts for the initial complaint in 75%. Approximately 80% of patients with ocular onset progress to involvement of other muscle groups (usually within 2 years), while 20% have only ocular complaints

    E.   Impaired neuromuscular transmission of myasthenia is due to the presence of antibodies to acetylcholine receptors in the motor endplate of striated muscles. This leads to a reduction in the number of acetylcholine receptors

    F.   Clinical characteristics of ocular myasthenia:

        1.   Variability of muscle function within minutes, hours, days, or weeks

        2.   Remissions and exacerbations (often triggered by infection or trauma)

        3.   Onset at any age

        4.   Ptosis (unilateral or bilateral) worse at end of day, may "shift" from eye to eye

        5.   Extraocular muscle involvement follows no set pattern; any ocular movement pattern may develop and thus mimic any ocular motor cranial nerve palsy or central gaze disturbance (eg, gaze palsy, internuclear ophthalmoplegia, gaze-evoked nystagmus)

      6.   Dysthyroidism is found in approximately 5% of myasthenics, also an increased incidence of thymoma and collagen vascular disorders

G.   Diagnosis of ocular myasthenia

    1.   Lid fatigue: with sustained upward gaze ptosis, becomes more marked

    2.   Lid-twitch sign (Cogan): the patient looks down for 10 to 15 seconds and is then asked to rapidly refixate in the primary position. A positive lid-twitch sign consists of an upward overshoot of the lid, which then falls to its previously ptotic position

    3.   Enhanced ptosis: if ptosis is asymmetric, the patient may use the frontalis muscle to elevate both lids, producing what appears to be lid retraction on one side. If the more ptotic lid is elevated, the previously retracted one will fall

    4.   Variability in measuring phorias or tropias during the same examination or at different times is very suggestive of myasthenia

    5.   Myasthenic ptosis is frequently associated with orbicularis weakness

    6.   Tensilon (edrophonium chloride) test: one positive test establishes the diagnosis of myasthenia, yet myasthenia may exist even in the face of a negative Tensilon test (see Chapter 20 for correct way to perform a Tensilon test)

    7.   **Alert!** Rarely:

        a.   Patient may have false-positive Tensilon test, or

        b.   Positive Tensilon test and coexistent intracranial mass (patient has two diseases)

    8.   Sleep test

        a.   Safe alternative to Tensilon test

        b.   Resolution of ptosis or ophthalmoparesis after 30-minute period of sleep, with reappearance of sign 30 seconds to 5 minutes after awakening

    9.   Ice test

        a.   Also safe alternative to Tensilon test

        b.   Resolution of ptosis after 2-minute application of ice pack to involved eyelid

        c.   High degree of sensitivity and specificity for myasthenic ptosis

    10.   Acetylcholine receptor antibodies, if present, are diagnostic of myasthenia. However, only about 60% of patients with ocular myasthenia have detectable antibody levels

    11.   Electromyography (EMG): with repetitive supramaximal motor nerve stimulation there is a decremental muscular response in myasthenia. Helpful if present, but may be a normal response in clinically uninvolved extremity musculature in patients with ocular myasthenia. Should be performed on orbicularis oculi as well

H.   Certain drugs may cause:

    1.   Unmasking or aggravation of myasthenia (eg, quinidine, propranolol, lithium)

    2.   Further impairment of neuromuscular conduction—aminoglycosides

    3.   Drug-induced myasthenia syndrome (eg, penicillamine)

I.   Treatment of ocular myasthenia

1. Occlusion of one eye
2. Prism spectacles
3. Pyridostigmine (Mestinon [Valeant Pharmaceuticals International, Aliso Viejo, Calif])
4. Systemic steroids

J. Treatment of systemic myasthenia
1. Pyridostigmine (Mestinon)
2. Immunosuppressants (steroids, cyclosporine, azathioprine)
3. Plasmapheresis
4. IV immune globulin (Ig)
5. Thymectomy

III. Chronic progressive external ophthalmoplegia (CPEO)

A. Comprises a group of disorders characterized by insidiously progressive, symmetric immobility of the eyes, with lids typically ptotic, the orbicularis oculi weak, and the pupils spared

B. The eye movements remain limited with doll's head and caloric stimulation

C. CPEO may occur in an isolated ocular form, may have a hereditary pattern, or may be part of a recognizable clinical entity
1. Oculopharyngeal dystrophy: dysphagia, family history of ophthalmoplegia, often of French-Canadian ancestry
2. Kearns-Sayre syndrome: triad of CPEO, cardiac conduction defect, pigmentary retinopathy
3. Ophthalmoplegia plus: term applied to instances in which CPEO is associated with the above abnormalities plus a variety of others, including elevated cerebrospinal fluid protein, spongiform degeneration of the cerebrum and brainstem, slow electroencephalogram (EEG), subnormal intelligence, hearing loss

D. Muscle biopsy (ocular or limb) will demonstrate mitochondrial accumulations beneath the plasma membrane and between myofibrils. Using a modified trichrome stain, these abnormal muscle fibers have been called "ragged red" fibers

E. CPEO in itself or as part of a multisystem disease may be associated with deletions in the mitochondrial DNA of skeletal muscle ("mitochondrial myopathy")

F. A condition simulating CPEO is known as Progressive Supranuclear Palsy or Steele-Richardson-Olszewski syndrome
1. Vertical gaze is affected first often with slowing of vertical saccades and paresis of downward gaze
2. Eventually horizontal gaze is involved
3. Doll's head and caloric testing demonstrate full excursions until late in course of disease
4. Additional clinical findings: dystonic rigidity of neck and trunk, masked face, dysarthria, dysesthesia, hyperreflexia, dementia, apraxia of eyelid opening
5. Neurodegenerative condition characterized pathologically by neuronal loss, gliosis, neurofibrillary tangles, and demyelination centered in the brainstem reticular formation and ocular motor nuclei

6. Characterized by abnormal accumulation of microtubule-association protein, tau

7. Therapy: none of proven efficacy

IV. Myotonic dystrophy

A. Autosomal dominant muscular dystrophy in which myotonia is accompanied by dystrophic changes in other tissues and organs

B. Two genetic loci have been associated with the clinical phenotype: chromosome 19 (DM1) and chromosome 3 (DM2)

C. Myotonia is a phenomenon in which muscle fibers have a pathologically persistent activity after a strong contraction or are continuously active when they should be relaxed

D. Ophthalmologic signs
1. Bilateral ptosis
2. Progressive external ophthalmoplegia
3. Myotonia of lid closure and gaze holding
4. Orbicularis weaknesses
5. Polychromatophilic cataracts
6. Miotic pupils, sluggish to light and near
7. Retinal pigmentary degeneration

E. Multiple systemic findings include face, neck, and limb myopathy with atrophy, testicular atrophy, baldness, cardiac conduction defects

V. Dysthyroid myopathy (Graves' disease)

A. A restrictive myopathy occurring commonly in middle-aged and elderly individuals, leading to ophthalmoparesis and diplopia

B. Lymphocytic and plasmacytic infiltration of extraocular muscles; leads to edema, activation of fibroblasts with production of acid mucopolysaccharide and fibrosis

C. Variety of ocular motility patterns produced
1. "Elevator palsy" due to fibrotic shortening of the inferior rectus
2. "Abduction weaknesses" due to involvement of the medial rectus, mimicking a VI nerve palsy
3. Superior and lateral rectus muscles less frequently involved
4. Frequency of clinical involvement of rectus muscles: IR > MR > SR > LR

D. Additional findings include:
1. Proptosis
2. Lids: retraction, lid lag on downward gaze (von Graefe's sign), edema
3. Conjunctiva: injection over horizontal rectus muscles, chemosis
4. Cornea: keratopathy, erosions, ulceration
5. Optic neuropathy due to compression at orbital apex by enlarged extraocular muscles (see Chapter 9, VII, A, 3)

E. Table 11-1 summarizes clinical findings with "NO SPECS" mnemonic classification and soft-tissue involvement with "RELIEF" mnemonic

F. Diagnostic studies
1. Forced duction testing (see Chapter 20)

Table 11-1

GRAVES' DISEASE SIGNS (MNEMONIC)

No signs or symptoms
Only signs of lid retraction, lid lag, stare
Soft tissue signs and symptoms:
    Resistance to retropulsion
    Edema of conjunctiva and caruncle
    Lacrimal gland enlargement
    Injection over rectus muscle insertion
    Edema of eyelids
    Fullness of eyelids
Proptosis
Extraocular muscle enlargement
Corneal exposure secondary to exposure
Sight loss secondary to optic nerve compression

Modified from Van Dyk HJ. Orbital Graves' disease. A modification of the NO SPECS classification. *Ophthalmology.* 1981;88:479-483.

2. Ultrasonography to measure size of extraocular muscles
3. Orbital computed tomography (CT) scanning
    a. Typically enlargement of all extraocular muscles in both orbits
    b. Muscle tendon spared
4. Thyroid function tests

G. Association of dysthyroidism with myasthenia; two diseases may coexist and give a variety of ocular findings

VI. Idiopathic orbital inflammation (orbital pseudotumor)

A. A syndrome occurring in any age group consisting of acute onset of orbital pain, chemosis, conjunctival injection, and frequently proptosis

B. If the inflammatory process affects one or more of the extraocular muscles, the term orbital myositis is employed. These patients typically complain of diplopia

C. Pathologic studies in such cases demonstrate orbital structures (blood vessels, muscles, lacrimal glands, etc) infiltrated with chronic inflammatory cells

D. In the vast majority of cases, the etiology of the inflammatory response is unknown, although it may occur with systemic disorders, including lupus erythematosus, rheumatoid arthritis, sarcoidosis, Wegener's granulomatosis, dermatomyositis

E. Diagnostic studies
1. Orbital ultrasonography
2. Orbital CT scanning
    a. Usually only one or two extraocular muscles enlarged in a single orbit (myositis)

b.   Muscle tendon enlarged as well
3.   Orbital biopsy

F.   Intracranial spread occurs in 5% to 10% of cases; patient may or may not have symptoms of central nervous system involvement

G.   Treatment modalities
1.   Systemic steroids usually produce dramatic improvement in symptoms in 24 to 48 hours with clearing of signs over 1 to 4 weeks
2.   Orbital radiation therapy: 1000 to 2000 cGy
3.   Chlorambucil, cyclophosphamide, or cyclosporine for chronic, recurrent orbital pseudotumor

H.   It may be difficult to distinguish between idiopathic orbital inflammation and orbital lymphoma, both clinically and pathologically. All patients with idiopathic orbital inflammation must be followed carefully. An initial salutary response to steroid therapy by no means excludes a malignant process

BIBLIOGRAPHY

Books

Char DH. *Thyroid Eye Disease*. 3rd ed. New York, NY: Butterworth-Heinemann; 1997.

Lisak RP, Barchi RL. *Myasthenia Gravis and Myasthenic Syndromes*. New York, NY: Marcel Dekker; 1994.

Rootman J. *Diseases of the Orbit*. 3rd ed. Philadelphia, Pa: Lippincott Williams & Wilkins; 2003.

Chapters

Calvert PC. Disorders of neuromuscular transmission. In: Miller NR, Newman NJ, eds. *Walsh and Hoyt's Clinical Neuro-Ophthalmology*. 6th ed. Vol 1. Philadelphia, Pa: Lippincott Williams & Wilkins; 2005:1041-1084.

Glaser JS, Siatkowski RM. Infranuclear disorders of eye movement. In: Glaser JS, ed. *Neuro-Ophthalmology*. 3rd ed. Philadelphia, Pa: Lippincott Williams & Wilkins; 1999:405-460.

Hoffman PN. Myopathies affecting the extraocular muscles. In: Miller NR, Newman NJ, eds. *Walsh and Hoyt's Clinical Neuro-Ophthalmology*. 6th ed. Vol 1. Philadelphia, Pa: Lippincott Williams & Wilkins; 2005:1085-1131.

Articles

Cogan DG. Myasthenia gravis: a review of the disease and a description of lid twitch as a characteristic sign. *Arch Ophthalmol*. 1965;74:217-221.

Conti-Fine BM, Milani M, Kaminski HJ. Myasthenia gravis: past, present, and future. *J Clin Invest*. 2006;116:2843-2854.

Drachman DA. Ophthalmoplegia plus: the neuro-degenerative disorders associated with progressive external ophthalmoplegia. *Arch Neurol*. 1968;18:654-674.

Elrod RD, Weinberg DA. Ocular myasthenia gravis. *Ophthalmol Clin North Am*. 2004;17:275-309.

Glaser JS. Myasthenic pseudo-internuclear ophthalmoplegia. *Arch Ophthalmol*. 1966;75:363-366.

Gorelick PB, Pena R, Lee AG, et al. An ice test for the diagnosis of myasthenia gravis. *Ophthalmology*. 1999;106:1282-1286.

Gorman CA, Garrity JA, Fatourechi V, et al. A prospective, randomized, double-blind, placebo-controlled study of orbital radiotherapy for Graves' ophthalmopathy. *Ophthalmology*. 2001;108:1523-1534.

Kazim M, Goldberg RA, Smith TJ. Insights into the pathogenesis of thyroid-associated orbitopathy. *Arch Ophthalmol*. 2002;120:380-388.

Kearns TB, Sayre GP. Retinitis pigmentosa, external ophthalmoplegia and complete heart block. *Arch Ophthalmol*. 1958;60:280-289.

Mahr MA, Salomao DR, Garrity JA. Inflammatory orbital pseudotumor with extension beyond the orbit. *Am J Ophthalmol*. 2004;138:396-400.

Newman NJ. Mitochondrial diseases and the eye. *Ophthalmol Clin North Am*. 1992;5:405-424.

Odel JG, Winterkorn JMS, Behrens MM. The sleep test for myasthenia gravis. *Journal of Clinical Neuro-Ophthalmology*. 1991;11:288-292.

Osserman KE, Kaplan LI. Rapid diagnostic test for myasthenia gravis: increased muscle strength, without fasciculations, after intravenous administration of edrophonium (Tensilon) chloride. *JAMA*. 1952;150:265-269.

Rampello L, Butta V, Raffaele R, et al. Progressive supranuclear palsy: a systematic review. *Neurobiol Dis*. 2005;20:179-186.

Sanders DB, Andrews PI, Howard JF, et al. Seronegative myasthenia gravis. *Neurology*. 1997;48(Suppl S):S40-S45.

Spoor TC, Martinez AJ, Kennerdell JS, et al. Dysthyroid and myasthenia myopathy of the medial rectus: a clinical pathologic report. *Neurology*. 1980;30:939-944.

Steele JC, Richardson JC, Olsewski J. Progressive supranuclear palsy. *Arch Neurol*. 1964;10:333-359.

Chapter 12

V Nerve (Trigeminal) Syndromes

Lanning B. Kline, MD

I. **Anatomical considerations (Figure 12-1)**

    A.   The trigeminal nerve is a mixed nerve

        1.   Sensory—ipsilateral side of face

        2.   Motor—ipsilateral muscles of mastication (masseter, temporalis, pterygoids)

    B.   Nuclear complex

        1.   Sensory portion of trigeminal nerve extends from the midbrain to the upper cervical cord

        2.   Mesencephalic (rostral) nucleus—proprioception and deep sensation from tendons and muscles of mastication

        3.   Main sensory nucleus

            a.   Located in pons

            b.   Subserves light touch

        4.   Spinal nucleus

            a.   Extends from pons to upper cervical cord

            b.   Subserves pain and temperature

            c.   Divided into segments that correspond to dermatomes that are concentric around the mouth

    C.   Peripheral nerve

        1.   The trigeminal nerve supplies sensation to the ipsilateral side of the face via three branches

            a. V^1—Ophthalmic division: frontal, lacrimal, and nasociliary

            b. V^2—Maxillary division: cheek and lower eyelid

            c. V^3—Mandibular division: area of mandible (but not angle of mandible), lower lip, tongue

        2.   Motor nucleus lies in pons medially to main sensory nucleus and axons travel with mandibular (V^3) division

        3.   Three divisions of trigeminal nerve converge at trigeminal (gasserian) ganglion, which lies in Meckel's cave of temporal bone

        4.   Fibers then travel through main sensory root to brainstem

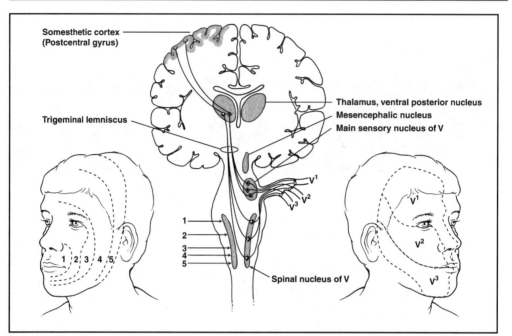

Figure 12-1. Diagram of the central pathways and peripheral innervation of the V nerve.

II. Oculofacial hypesthesia (see Figure 12-1)

A. Distribution of facial numbness or paresthesias helps determine central or peripheral origin

1. Concentric perioral numbness/paresthesia—central (nuclear) origin (eg, ischemia, demyelination)

2. Band of numbness/paresthesia—peripheral origin (ie, V^1, V^2, V^3)

3. Such somatotopic hypesthesia (eg, V^1 only, or V^2 and V^3 with sparing of V^1) suggests that the lesion is more likely to be in the middle cranial fossa (cavernous sinus) or orbit

B. Differential diagnosis of diminished sensation in the trigeminal distribution (Glaser, 1999)

1. Corneal
   a. Herpes simplex
   b. Herpes zoster
   c. Ocular surgery
   d. Cerebellopontine angle tumors
   e. Dysautonomia
   f. Congenital

2. Ophthalmic division
   a. Neoplasm, orbital apex
   b. Neoplasm, superior orbital fissure
   c. Neoplasm, cavernous sinus
   d. Neoplasm, middle fossa
   e. Aneurysm, cavernous sinus

3. Maxillary division
   a. Orbit floor fracture
   b. Maxillary antrum carcinoma
   c. Perineural spread of skin carcinoma (see Chapter 12, III, B, 5)
   d. Neoplasm, foremen rotundum, sphenopterygoid fossa
4. Mandibular division
   a. Nasopharyngeal tumor
   b. Middle fossa tumor
   c. Numb chin syndrome
      i. Involvement of mental nerve (terminal branch of inferior alveolar nerve)
      ii. Frequently due to systemic cancer: breast, lymphoproliferative disorders
      iii. Contrast—enhanced imaging (computed tomography [CT] or magnetic resonance imaging [MRI]) of head including skull base and mandible
5. All divisions
   a. Nasopharyngeal carcinoma
   b. Cerebellopontine angle tumors
   c. Brainstem lesions (dissociated sensory loss)
   d. Intracavernous aneurysm
   e. Demyelinative
   f. Middle fossa or Meckel's cave tumor
   g. Benign sensory neuropathy
   h. Tentorial meningioma
   i. Toxins (eg, trichloroethylene)
   j. Trigeminal neurofibroma

III. Oculofacial pain

A. Differential diagnosis of relatively common entities associated with ocular and facial pain (Glaser, 1999)
   1. Ocular
      a. Local corneal, lid, and anterior segment disease
      b. Ocular inflammation
      c. Dry eye and tear deficiency syndromes
      d. Chronic ocular hypoxia, carotid occlusive disease
      e. Angle-closure glaucoma
   2. Ophthalmic division
      a. Migraine, cluster headaches
      b. Raeder's paratrigeminal neuralgia
      c. Painful ophthalmoplegia syndromes
      d. Herpes zoster—nasociliary nerve involvement indicated by vesicular eruption on side or tip of nose (Hutchison's sign)
      e. Referred (dural) pain, including occipital infarction
      f. Tic douloureux (infrequent in V^1)
      g. Sinusitis

3. Maxillary division
   a. Tic douloureux
   b. Nasopharyngeal carcinoma
   c. Temporomandibular syndrome
   d. Dental disease
   e. Sinusitis
4. Mandibular division
   a. Tic douloureux
   b. Dental disease
5. Miscellaneous
   a. Atypical facial neuralgias
   b. Pain with medullary lesions (eg, Wallenberg syndrome)
   c. Giant cell arteritis (see Chapter 9)
   d. Trigeminal tumors

B. Specific trigeminal syndromes
   1. Referred pain
      a. Any intracranial process irritating the dural sensory fibers, which may be supplied by recurrent branches of V nerve
      b. Neck pain (eg, from osteoarthritis in the cervical spine) may be referred to the eye because of the cervical sensory fibers traveling with the trigeminal fibers of the spinal tract of V, which extends to C-2 level
   2. Trigeminal neuralgia (tic douloureux)
      a. Paroxysmal pain in the distribution of one or more of the divisions of V ($V^3 > V^2 > V^1$)
      b. Recurring, lancinating, "lightning" hemifacial pain lasting 20 to 30 seconds
      c. Pain may be so intense that the facial muscles contract and distort the face during an attack. Frequently "triggered" by touching certain areas of the face or scalp; asymptomatic or mild headache between episodes
      d. No neurologic deficits (including normal corneal reflex)
      e. Neuralgia of more persistent nature and associated with neurologic deficits may resolve from compressive, demyelinative, or inflammatory lesion of the V nerve
   3. Herpetic neuralgia
      a. Pain of herpes zoster is described as severe, burning, aching in quality
      b. Pain occurs over distribution of a dermatome of cranial nerve, usually V^1, although it may involve the facial nerve (external ear) with ipsilateral facial palsy (Ramsay Hunt syndrome)
      c. Pain often precedes onset of typical rash by 4 to 7 days
      d. Pain usually regresses within 1 to 2 weeks, but may persist for months or years: post-herpetic neuralgia
      e. Patients typically describe dysesthesias as "crawling" and "prickly" sensations
   4. Raeder's paratrigeminal neuralgia
      a. V nerve distribution pain with ipsilateral Horner's syndrome

      b. Almost exclusively in middle-aged or elderly male patients

      c. May be caused by migrainous dilation of the internal carotid artery with compression of the V nerve and sympathetic plexus in the middle cranial fossa

      d. If the pain is persistent (not of migrainous episodic nature) or if associated with cranial nerve palsy, then suspect a middle fossa tumor, aneurysm, or internal carotid artery dissection

5. Perineural spread of cancer

      a. Initial involvement often limited to single nerve branch (especially infraorbital) but proximal spread leads to cavernous sinus involvement

      b. Often signals recurrence of previously treated tumor

      c. Frequently due to squamous cell carcinoma of the face or oropharyngeal mucosa

      d. Diagnosis established with contrast-enhanced MRI

BIBLIOGRAPHY

Books

Fromm GH, Sessle BJ. *Trigeminal Neuralgia: Current Concepts Regarding Pathogenesis and Treatment.* Boston, Mass: Butterworth-Heinemann; 1991.

Chapters

Glaser JS. *Neuro-Ophthalmology.* 3rd ed. Philadelphia, Pa: Lippincott Williams & Wilkins; 1999:64-70.

Lavin PJM. Ocular and facial pain syndromes. In: Rosen ES, Eustace P, Thompson HS, Cumming WJK, eds. *Neuro-Ophthalmology.* St Louis, Mo: Mosby; 1998:1-18.

Liu GT. The trigeminal nerve and its central connections. In: Miller NR, Newman NJ, eds. *Walsh and Hoyt's Clinical Neuro-Ophthalmology.* 6th ed. Vol 1. Philadelphia, Pa: Lippincott Williams & Wilkins; 2005:1233-1274.

Martin TJ, Corbett JJ. *Neuro-Ophthalmology—The Requisites.* St Louis, Mo: Mosby; 2000:223-232.

Van Stavern GP. Headache and facial pain. In: Miller NR, Newman NJ, eds. *Walsh and Hoyt's Clinical Neuro-Ophthalmology.* 6th ed. Vol 1. Philadelphia, Pa: Lippincott Williams & Wilkins; 2005:1275-1311.

Articles

Biousse V, Toubol PJ, D'Anglejan–Chatillon J, et al. Ophthalmologic manifestation of internal carotid artery dissection. *Am J Ophthalmol.* 1998;126:565-577.

Clouston PD, Sharpe DM, Corbett AJ, et al. Perineural spread of cutaneous head and neck cancer: its orbital and central neurologic complications. *Arch Neurol.* 1990;47:73-77.

Feindel W, Penfield W, McNaughton F. The tentorial nerves and localization of intracranial pain in man. *Neurology.* 1960;10:555-563.

Kust RG, Straus SE. Postherpetic neuralgia: pathogenesis, treatment and prevention. *N Engl J Med.* 1996;335:32-42.

Lossos A, Siegal T. Numb chin syndrome in cancer patients: etiology response to treatment and prognostic significance. *Neurology.* 1992;70:877-881.

Chapter 13

The Seven Syndromes of the VII Nerve (Facial)

Lanning B. Kline, MD

I. **Anatomical considerations**

    A.   Figure 13-1 is a schematic representation of the course of the supranuclear and infranuclear fibers controlling the facial musculature. The fibers are accompanied by the nervus intermedius (tearing, salivation, taste), as well as sensory fibers from the external ear and the nerve to the stapedius muscle. The nerve leaves the pons and travels with the VIII cranial nerve through the internal auditory canal, leaving the canal through the fallopian canal, which courses inferiorly through the petrous bone, exiting through the stylomastoid foramen

II. **The seven syndromes of the VII nerve**

    A.   Supranuclear facial palsy (see Figure 13-1, site 1) results in contralateral weakness of the lower two thirds of the face, with some weakness of the orbicularis oculi, but not as severe as with peripheral VII nerve palsy (Figures 13-2a and 13-2b); does not usually require tarsorrhaphy

    B.   Recent anatomic studies in the primate suggest an alternate explanation for sparing of the upper one third of the face with an upper motor neuron lesion: one subsector of the facial nucleus (M3 or rostral cingulate motor region) provides bilateral innervation to the upper facial region (Morecraft, 2001)

    C.   Cerebellopontine angle tumor (see Figure 13-1, site 2)

        1.   Total ipsilateral facial weakness

        2.   Decreased tearing (nervus intermedius)

        3.   Hyperacusis (nerve to stapedius muscle)

        4.   Decreased taste of anterior two thirds of tongue (nervus intermedius and chorda tympani)

        5.   Associated neurologic deficits: V, VI, VIII, Horner's syndrome, gaze palsy, nystagmus, papilledema, cerebellar dysfunction

    D.   Geniculate ganglionitis (Ramsay Hunt syndrome, zoster oticus [see Figure 13-1, site 3])

        1.   Same findings as Figure 13-1, site 2; no associated neurologic deficits except for possibly a VIII nerve involvement (hearing loss, vestibular dysfunction)

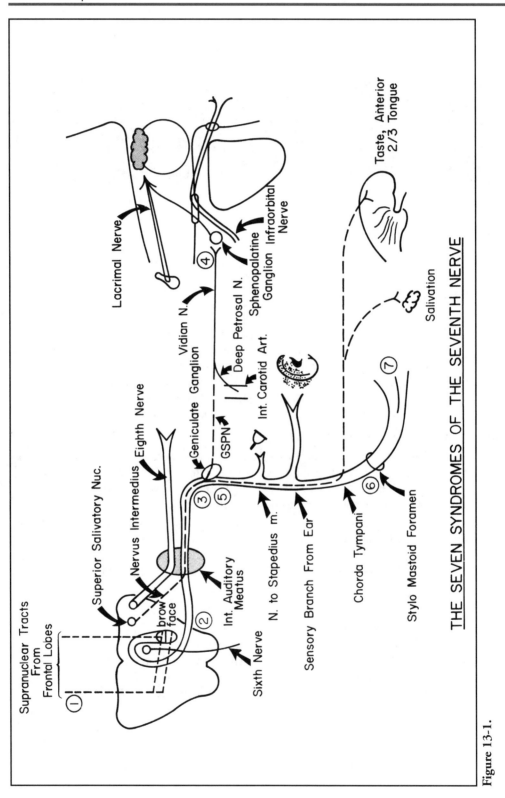

THE SEVEN SYNDROMES OF THE SEVENTH NERVE

Taste, Anterior 2/3 Tongue

Salivation

Lacrimal Nerve

Sphenopalatine Ganglion Infraorbital Nerve

Deep Petrosal N.

Vidian N.

Int. Carotid Art.

Geniculate Ganglion

GSPN

Eighth Nerve

Nervus Intermedius

Superior Salivatory Nuc.

Supranuclear Tracts From Frontal Lobes

brow
face

Int. Auditory Meatus

Sixth Nerve

N. to Stapedius m.

Sensory Branch From Ear

Chorda Tympani

Stylo Mastoid Foramen

Figure 13-1.

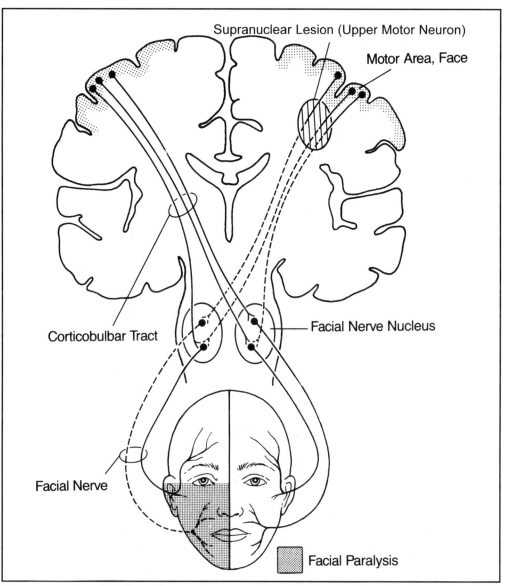

Figure 13-2a. Facial weakness due to an upper motor neuron lesion.

    2.   May see zoster vesicles in areas supplied by sensory portion of VII nerve: tympanic membrane, external auditory canal, pinna, buccal mucosa, neck

    3.   Recovery is poorer than with Bell's palsy (see below)

E.   Isolated ipsilateral tear deficiency (see Figure 13-1, site 4)

    1.   Nasopharyngeal carcinoma may affect the vidian nerve or sphenopalatine ganglion; often accompanying VI nerve palsy due to cavernous sinus involvement

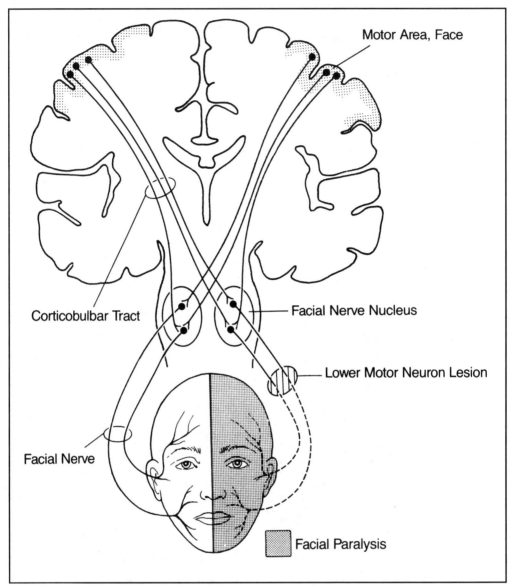

Figure 13-2b. Facial weakness due to a lower motor neuron lesion.

F. Bell's palsy (see Figure 13-1, site 5)
    1. Common idiopathic facial palsy, possibly due to viral infection and edema of VII nerve within fallopian canal
    2. Same findings as Figure 13-1, site 2 except for no associated neurologic deficits; tearing may be normal
    3. Complete recovery, within 60 days in 75% of patients; with steroid therapy, recovery over 90%
    4. Antiviral agents often used: acyclovir, famciclovir
G. Isolated total ipsilateral facial palsy (see Figure 13-1, site 6)

       1.   Mastoidopathy, facial trauma, parotid gland surgery

  H.   Isolated partial ipsilateral facial palsy (see Figure 13-1, site 7)

       1.   Only certain branches of VII nerve are affected

III. Facial diplegia

  A.   Brainstem contusion

  B.   Brainstem stroke (basilar artery)

  C.   Brainstem glioma

  D.   Möbius syndrome: aplasia of VII nerve nuclei in brainstem; often accompanied by:

       1.   Bilateral VI nerve palsies

       2.   Palatal and lingual palsy

       3.   Deafness

       4.   Deficiencies of pectoral and lingual muscles

       5.   Extremity defects: syndactyly, supernumerary digits, absent fingers and toes

       6.   Rarely inherited; defect on chromosome 3q

  E.   Myasthenia gravis (see Chapter 11)

  F.   Guillain-Barré syndrome

       1.   Autoimmune acute peripheral neuropathy

       2.   Subtypes:

           a.   Acute inflammatory demyelinating polyneuropathy (AIDP)

               i.   Motor weakness, often ascending which progresses up to 4 weeks

               ii.   Frequently preceded by flu-like episode or gastroenteritis

               iii. One half of patients develop unilateral or bilateral facial weakness

               iv. Ophthalmoplegia

               v.   Ptosis

               vi. Optic nerve involvement: papilledema (with very high cerebrospinal fluid [CSF] protein); optic neuritis

               vii. CSF: albuminocytologic dissociation (elevated protein without pleocytosis)

               viii. Treatment: plasma exchange; IV immunoglobulin (Ig)

           b.   Miller Fisher syndrome (see Chapter 7, V, G)

  G.   Myotonic dystrophy (see Chapter 11, IV)

  H.   Melkersson-Rosenthal syndrome

       1.   Rare, idiopathic disorder

       2.   Facial swelling

       3.   Transversely fissured tongue

       4.   Recurrent, alternating facial palsy

  I.   Neoplastic: leukemia, meningeal carcinomatosis

  J.   Inflammatory: sarcoidosis, porphyria

  K.   Infectious: polio, AIDS, Lyme disease

IV. Crocodile tears (gustolacrimal reflex)

    A.   Any patient with VII nerve palsy that has affected the parasympathetic fibers stimulating tearing and salivation may experience tearing at mealtime due to aberrant regeneration or misdirection of fibers, so that when neural stimulus for salivation is transmitted, it results in stimulation of tearing

V. Spastic paretic facial contracture (see Chapter 14, V, C, 5)

    A.   Unilateral spastic facial contracture with associated facial weakness

    B.   May be indicative of intrinsic pontine disease (neoplasm, stroke, multiple sclerosis)

    C.   Due to damage of VII nerve nucleus (facial paresis) and its supranuclear connections (facial spasticity)

    D.   Other causes include extra-axial compression (cerebellopontine angle mass), Bell's palsy, Guillain-Barré syndrome

VI. Blepharospasm

    A.   Onset usually in adult life (sixth and seventh decade); 3:1 female predominance

    B.   Bilateral, episodic, involuntary contractions of the orbicularis oculi

    C.   At times, associated with involuntary spasm of the lower facial musculature: orofacial dyskinesia or Meige's syndrome

    D.   Etiology
        1.   Adults
            a.   Usually unknown ("essential" blepharospasm); possibly related to dysfunction of the basal ganglia and limbic system
            b.   May occur in patients with Parkinson's disease, progressive supranuclear palsy, Huntington's disease, multiple sclerosis, and brainstem stroke
        2.   Children
            a.   Usually benign, self-limited habit
            b.   Tourette's syndrome

    E.   Treatment
        1.   Pharmacologic: clonazepam (Klonopin [Roche Pharmaceuticals, Nutley, NJ])
        2.   Chemodenervation: botulinum toxin
        3.   Surgery: selective VII nerve sectioning; orbicularis myectomies

VII. Hemifacial spasm

    A.   Unilateral (rarely bilateral) spasm involving half of facial muscles, typically lasting several minutes at a time; persists during sleep

    B.   Painless, no sensory loss

    C.   Etiology
        1.   Aberrant vascular loop (dolichoectasia) compressing VII nerve in subarachnoid space where it exits the pons
        2.   Following Bell's palsy (postparalytic hemifacial spasm)

    D.   Treatment
        1.   Pharmacologic: carbamazepine, baclofen, clonazepam, neurontin
        2.   Chemodenervation: botulinum toxin
        3.   Surgery: posterior fossa craniotomy with insertion of inert material between vascular loop and VII nerve

VIII. Facial myokymia

    A.   Usually benign, self-limited

    B.   If persistent over weeks or months, then consider:

        1.   Multiple sclerosis

        2.   Brainstem glioma

        3.   Brainstem stroke

BIBLIOGRAPHY

Books

Brin MF, Hallett M, Jankovic J. *Scientific and Therapeutic Aspects of Botulinum Toxin*. Philadelphia, Pa: Lippincott Williams & Wilkins; 2002.

Chapters

Galetta S, May M. The facial nerve and related disorders of the face. In: Glaser JS, ed. *Neuro-Ophthalmology*. 3rd ed. Philadelphia, Pa: Lippincott Williams & Wilkins; 1999:293-326.

Liu GT, Volpe NJ, Galetta SL. *Neuro-Ophthalmology: Diagnosis and Management*. St Louis, Mo: WB Saunders; 2001:464-512.

Articles

Adour KK, Ruboyianes JM, van Doerston PG, et al. Bell's palsy treatment with acyclovir and prednisone compared with prednisone alone: a double-blind, randomized, controlled trial. *Ann Otol Rhinol Laryngol*. 1996;105:371-378.

Bauer CA, Coker NJ. Update on facial nerve disorders. *Otolaryngol Clin North Am*. 1996;29:445-454.

Hughes RA, Cornblath DR. Guillain-Barré syndrome. *Lancet*. 2005;366:1653-1666.

Jannetta PJ. The cause of hemifacial spasm: definitive microsurgical treatment at the brainstem in 31 patients. *Transactions of the American Academy of Ophthalmology and Otolaryngology*. 1974;80:319-322.

Morecraft RJ, Lovie JL, Herrick JL, et al. Cortical innervation of the facial nucleus in the non-human primate. *Brain*. 2001;124:176-208.

Steiner I, Maltan Y. Bell's palsy and herpes virus: to acyclovir or not to acyclovir. *J Neurol Sci*. 1999;170:19-23.

Chapter 14

Eyelid Disorders

Saunders L. Hupp, MD, and Jennifer T. Scruggs, MD

I. **Anatomical considerations (Figure 14-1)**

    A.   Eyelid opening (retraction) is mediated through

        1.   Levator palpebrae: primary elevator of upper eyelid

        2.   Muller's muscle: secondary elevator of upper eyelid

            a.   Corresponding muscle in lower eyelid is known as inferior tarsal muscle

        3.   Frontalis muscle: secondary elevator of upper eyelid

    B.   Eyelid closing (protraction) is mediated through

        1.   Orbicularis oculi: primary closure of upper and lower lids

        2.   Procerus muscle: secondary closure of upper eyelid

        3.   Corrugator muscle: secondary closure of upper eyelid

    C.   Innervation of eyelid opening

        1.   Levator palpebrae: superior division of III nerve (see Figure 5-1)

        2.   Muller's muscle (and inferior tarsal muscle): oculosympathetic pathway, third order neuron (see Figure 8-3)

        3.   Frontalis muscle: VII nerve

    D.   Innervation of eyelid closing

        1.   Orbicularis oculi: VII nerve (see Figures 13-2a and 13-2b)

        2.   Procerus muscle: VII nerve

        3.   Corrugator muscle: VII nerve

II. **Physiology of eyelid opening**

    A.   Supranuclear control of eyelid opening

        1.   Through both corticobulbar and extrapyramidal pathways

        2.   Areas of the frontal, occipital, and temporal cortex have been associated with eyelid opening

        3.   Arousal state of the brain influences palpebral fissure width through control of levator tonus

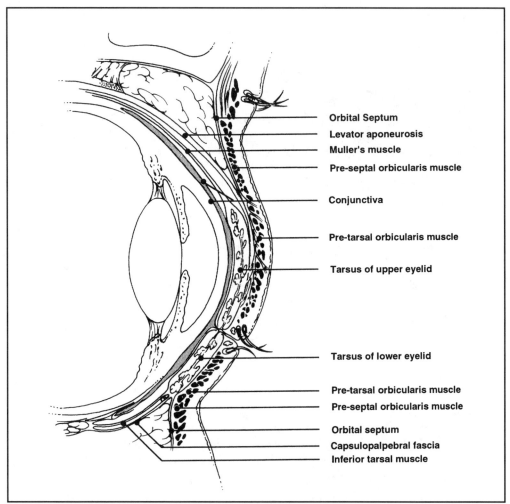

Orbital Septum
Levator aponeurosis
Muller's muscle
Pre-septal orbicularis muscle

Conjunctiva

Pre-tarsal orbicularis muscle

Tarsus of upper eyelid

Tarsus of lower eyelid

Pre-tarsal orbicularis muscle
Pre-septal orbicularis muscle

Orbital septum
Capsulopalpebral fascia
Inferior tarsal muscle

Figure 14-1. Anatomy of the upper and lower eyelids.

B.   Final common pathway for eyelid opening
  1.   Central caudal subnucleus of III nerve nuclear complex to both levator palpebrae muscles
  2.   Nerve fibers to the levator muscle travel with the superior division of III nerve
C.   Physiologic synkineses link the activity of the levator muscles to related extraocular and facial muscle movement
  1.   Movements of the upper eyelids are identically coordinated, obeying Hering's law of equal innervation: the eyelids lift with upgaze and lower with downgaze
  2.   Voluntary reflex blinking: inhibition of levator tonus occurs with stimulation of the VII nerve

III.   Abnormalities of eyelid opening

A. Ptosis (blepharoptosis)—insufficient eyelid opening from drooping of the upper eyelid. Ptosis may be congenital or acquired. Classification is based on etiology

  1. Myogenic ptosis—results from an abnormal levator muscle; may be congenital or acquired

    a. Typical features

      i. Poor levator function (<5 mm)

      ii. Poorly defined or absent upper lid crease

      iii. Poorly defined upper lid superior sulcus

      iv. Lagophthalmos on downgaze

    b. Congenital myogenic ptosis—results from a poorly developed levator muscle with replacement of muscle fibers by fat and fibrous tissue

      i. Accounts for most cases of congenital ptosis

      ii. May be unilateral or bilateral

      iii. Most commonly is an isolated finding

      iv. May have ocular or systemic associations

        a. Blepharophimosis syndrome—bilateral ptosis, horizontal phimosis of lid fissures, telecanthus, epicanthus inversus

        b. Congenital fibrosis of the extraocular muscles

        c. Superior rectus weakness (double elevator palsy)

        d. Coexistent strabismus or amblyopia

    c. Acquired myogenic ptosis—results from localized or diffuse muscular disease

      i. Rare cause of acquired ptosis

      ii. Commonly have ocular or systemic associations

        a. Chronic progressive external ophthalmoplegia (see Chapter 11)

        b. Muscular dystrophy

        c. Myotonic dystrophy (see Chapter 11)

        d. Oculopharyngeal dystrophy (see Chapter 11)

        e. Corticosteriod-induced ptosis

          1. May be a localized form of steroid myopathy from long-term corticosteroid therapy (uveitis)

  2. Aponeurotic ptosis—results from attenuation, dehiscence, or disinsertion of the levator aponeurosis from its normal insertion on the anterior tarsus. Levator muscle function is normal

    a. Most common type of ptosis; also know "involutional" ptosis

    b. Typical features

      i. Good levator function (>10 mm)

      ii. High upper lid crease

      iii. Deep upper lid superior sulcus

      iv. Lid position is lower in downgaze

    c. Contributing factors

      i. Aging

      ii. Chronic inflammation

      iii. Blunt trauma

        iv.   Repetitive traction on the lid (eye rubbing, rigid contact lens use)

        v.   Prior ophthalmic surgery

3.   Neurogenic ptosis—results from innervational defects to the elevators of the eyelid; may be congenital or acquired

    a.   Marcus Gunn jaw-winking phenomenon—a congenital synkinetic ptosis resulting from aberrant connections between the motor division of V nerve and III nerve

        i.   Most common synkinetic movement associated with congenital ptosis

        ii.   External pterygoid—levator synkinesis: elevation of lid with movement of mandible to opposite side, protruded forward, or wide opening of the mouth

        iii.   Internal pterygoid—levator synkinesis: elevation of the lid with clenching of the teeth

    b.   Horner's syndrome (see Chapter 8)—results from lesions of oculosympathetic pathway with paralysis of Muller's muscle

        i.   Ptosis is mild, usually less than 3 mm

        ii.   "Upside-down" ptosis of the lower lid: mild elevation of the lower lid with relaxation of the inferior tarsal muscle

    c.   III nerve palsy (see Chapter 5)—results from lesions of III nerve with paralysis of the levator muscle

        i.   Ptosis may be partial or complete

    d.   "Cortical ptosis"—results from interruption of supranuclear pathways from unilateral temporal, occipital, or bilateral frontal cortical lesions

        i.   Unilateral or bilateral ptosis

        ii.   Supranuclear ptosis may appear in patients with non-organic disease

    e.   Paradoxic supranuclear inhibition of levator tonus

        i.   Ptosis may be isolated or associated with congenital horizontal or vertical eye movement abnormalities

        ii.   Inverse Marcus Gunn phenomenon

            a.   Eyelid closure during mouth opening

            b.   With downward movement of the lower jaw, there is total inhibition of the levator with subsequent ptosis

    f.   Ophthalmoplegic migraine (see Chapter 15)

4.   Neuromuscular ptosis—results from abnormalities of the neuromuscular junction

    a.   Myasthenia gravis (see Chapter 11)—results from deficiency of acetylcholine receptors at the neuromuscular junction

        i.   Ptosis is the most common presenting sign; initial manifestation in up to 75% of patients

        ii.   Variable, typically worsens with fatigue

        iii.   May be produced by having the patient sustain upgaze

        iv.   Look for Cogan's lid twitch sign

        v.   Frequently associated with orbicularis weakness

        vi.   May be accompanied by ocular motility disturbances

          vii.   **Remember:** consider Tensilon testing in all patients with onset of acquired isolated ptosis

     b.   Botulism (see Chapter 7)

     c.   Iatrogenic periocular botulinum toxin injections

         i.   Transient ptosis from infiltration of toxin into levator

5.   Mechanical ptosis—results from excess weight of the lid that interferes with eyelid movement

     a.   Dermatochalasis

     b.   Brow ptosis

     c.   Edema from blunt trauma or inflammation

     d.   Eyelid tumors: hemangioma, neurofibroma, large chalazion, basal cell carcinoma, squamous cell carcinoma

     e.   Eyelid infiltration: amyloidosis, lymphoma

     f.   Anterior orbital tumors

     g.   Cicatricial: damage following surgery, chemical or thermal injury, or inflammation (trachoma, ocular pemphigoid)

6.   Traumatic ptosis—results from blunt or sharp trauma to levator muscle or aponeurosis

     a.   Blunt trauma with levator dehiscence

     b.   Lid laceration

     c.   Occult lid or orbital foreign body

     d.   Orbital roof fracture

7.   Pseudoptosis—results from abnormalities of ocular, orbital, or facial anatomy with insufficient posterior support of the eyelid

     a.   Enophthalmos

     b.   Phthisis bulbi

     c.   Microphthalmos or anophthalmos

     d.   Hypotropia

     e.   Contralateral lid retraction

8.   Remember Hering's law of equal innervation (to both levators):

     a.   With asymmetric ptosis, patient uses frontalis to elevate both lids—produces lid retraction on one side. With manual elevation (or use of phenylephrine drops to stimulate Muller's muscle) of the more ptotic lid, the previously retracted lid falls—phenomenon termed "enhanced ptosis"

B.   Lid retraction—excessive eyelid opening characterized by sclera visible above superior corneal limbus when the eyes are directed straight ahead (superior scleral show)

   1.   Myopathic lid retraction

     a.   Most common form of lid retraction due to thyroid eye disease

         i.   Lid retraction is the most common presenting sign of thyroid eye disease

         ii.   Congenital transient lid retraction may be associated with maternal hyperthyroidism

     b.   Sympathomimetic drops (phenylephrine) stimulate Muller's muscle

     c.   Hepatic cirrhosis

      d.   Maldevelopment of levator muscle

  2.   Neuropathic lid retraction

    a.   Supranuclear lid retraction

        i.   Often associated with lesions of the rostral dorsal midbrain in the region of the nucleus of the posterior commissure (Collier's sign)

        ii.   Combination of lid retraction with downward displacement of eyes in infants produces the "setting sun" sign

        iii.   Periodic lid retraction may occur as isolated myoclonic movement or as part of vertical nystagmus seen with ocular myoclonus (see Chapter 3)

        iv.   Comatose patient may demonstrate periodic lid retraction synchronous with breathing or head movements

    b.   Paradoxic levator excitation with lid retraction

        i.   Congenital lid retraction may be seen with abnormalities of horizontal gaze (Duane's syndrome), jaw movements (Marcus Gunn phenomenon), or swallowing

        ii.   Acquired lid retraction may be seen with aberrant regeneration following III nerve palsy (pseudo von Graefe's sign)

        iii.   Claude Bernard syndrome: irritative lesion of oculosympathetic pathway produces lid retraction and an enlarged ipsilateral pupil (opposite of Horner's syndrome)

  3.   Physiologic lid retraction—results from physiologic response (Hering's law) to ptosis of the contralateral eye

  4.   Eyelid lag—results from lack of inhibition of upper eyelids on downgaze

    a.   Most commonly associated with lid retraction due to thyroid eye disease

    b.   May occur without lid retraction in extrapyramidal syndromes with lesions of the midbrain involving the nucleus of the posterior commissure

        i.   Parkinson's disease

        ii.   Progressive supranuclear palsy

        iii.   Thalamic-midbrain infarction

  C.   Apraxia of lid opening—nonparalytic inability to open eyes at will following voluntary or involuntary lid closure; no visible orbicularis oculi contraction

    1.   May occur in isolation

    2.   Majority of cases associated with benign essential blepharospasm

    3.   Other associations: basal ganglia disease, Huntington's chorea, Parkinson's disease, progressive supranuclear palsy

    4.   Neuroanatomic basis and central pathophysiology unknown

    5.   Thought to be due to involuntary levator palpbral inhibition and/or pretarsal orbicularis oculi contraction

IV. Physiology of eyelid closure

  A.   Lid closure may be unilateral (wink) or bilateral (blink)

  B.   Supranuclear control of eyelid closure

    1.   Cortical control of lid closure via bilateral corticobulbar pathways with predominant innervation to contralateral side

Table 14-1

PHYSIOLOGIC SYNKINESES AND REFLEX BLINKING

Reflex	Clinical Examination
Orbicularis stress	Tap lateral orbicularis oculi
Corneal blink	Corneal touch (V^1 nerve)
Cochleopalpebral	Sudden noise
Auropalpebral	Stimulate external auditory canal
Palatal palpebral	Touch palate
Bright flash	Rapid exposure to bright light

    2.   Subcortical control is mediated through extrapyramidal pathways that are affected by emotional states and tension

        a.   Extrapyramidal control may be absent in infants or synchronized with mouth movements, such as sucking

C.   Final common pathway for eyelid closure via VII nerve to orbicularis oculi (see Figure 13-1)

D.   Physiologic synkineses provide inverse relationship between superior rectus and eyelid movement during sleep and with forced eyelid closure

    1.   Bell's phenomenon: globe movement up and out as lids close

E.   Normal or periodic blinking

    1.   With each blink, there is complete inhibition of the levator just prior (10 milliseconds) to the onset of contraction of orbicularis oculi

        a.   Indicates interconnections between the central caudal nucleus of III nerve and nucleus of VII nerve

    2.   12 to 16 per minute in relaxed state

    3.   Decreased with reading or concentration

    4.   Increased with emotion (anxiety or arousal)

    5.   Protects and nourishes avascular cornea

    6.   Facilitates eye movement (saccade) to change the direction of gaze

F.   Reflex blinking is mediated though a variety of physiologic synkineses (Table 14-1)

V.   Abnormalities of eyelid closure

A.   Insufficient eyelid closure

    1.   Neurogenic—results from innervational defects

        a.   Supranuclear facial palsy (see Chapter 13)

        b.   Peripheral VII nerve palsy (see Chapter 13)

            i.   Cerebellopontine angle tumor

            ii.   Idiopathic (Bell's palsy)

    2.   Myogenic—results from decreased orbicularis oculi function

        a.   Myasthenia gravis—"peek" phenomenon: after sustained lid closure, lid opening occurs due to orbicularis fatigue

        b.   Muscular dystrophy

        c.   Myotonic dystrophy (see Chapter 11)

        d.   Chronic progressive external ophthalmoplegia (see Chapter 11)

    3.   Iatrogenic

        a.   After surgery involving recession of the inferior rectus muscle

        b.   After blepharoplasty with excessive skin or orbicularis excision

B.   Decreased blink rate

    1.   Parkinson's disease

    2.   Thyroid eye disease

    3.   Progressive supranuclear palsy

    4.   Infants in first few months of life

C.   Excessive eyelid closure—pathologic blinking or blepharospasm

    1.   Supranuclear blepharospasm

        a.   Benign essential blepharospasm (see Chapter 13)

            i.   Bilateral, episodic, involuntary contractions of the orbicularis oculi, procerus, and corrugator muscles

        b.   Orofacial dyskinesia (Meige's syndrome)

        c.   Focal seizure

        d.   Reflex blepharospasm (post-stroke)

        e.   Response to ocular irritation

        f.   Associated with tardive dyskinesia

        g.   Post-encephalitis

        h.   Habit spasms and tics (eg, Tourette's syndrome)

        i.   Non-organic

    2.   Pathologic blinking may occur in brainstem disease associated with decreased eye movements

        a.   Blink facilitates saccade through a blink-saccade synkinesis

        b.   May occur in Huntington's chorea, Gaucher's disease, Parkinson's disease, congenital ocular motor apraxia

    3.   Primary brainstem disease

        a.   Stroke

        b.   Demyelinating disease

        c.   Trauma

    4.   Benign facial or eyelid myokymia

    5.   Spastic paretic facial contracture (see Chapter 13, V)

        a.   Facial myokymia with contracture plus weakness of facial muscles

        b.   Etiologies:

            i.   Intra-axial (pons): tumor, stroke, multiple sclerosis

            ii.   Extra-axial: cerebellopontine angle mass, Bell's palsy, Guillain-Barré syndrome

    6.   Peripheral VII disease

        a.   Hemifacial spasm (see Chapter 13, VII)

            i.   "Idiopathic"—high percentage of cases may be due to aberrant vascular loop of vertebral and/or basilar arteries with compression of dorsal root entry zone of VII nerve

            ii.   Postparalytic—following VII palsy

7. Neuromuscular disease
    a. Tetany
    b. Strychnine poisoning
    c. Tetanus (risus sardonicus)
8. Systemic disease
    a. Hypothyroidism
    b. Myotonic dystrophy (see Chapter 11)
    c. Hyperkalemic familial paralysis
    d. Chondrodystrophic dystonia (Schwartz-Jampel syndrome)

D. Eyelid nystagmus
    1. Rhythmic oscillation of eyelids with a slow downward drift and a rapid upward phase
    2. Usually associated with:
        a. Convergence—seen in multiple sclerosis, Miller Fisher syndrome, brainstem lesion
        b. Gaze shifts—damage to brainstem or cerebellum
        c. Vertical nystagmus (eg, convergence-retraction nystagmus of dorsal midbrain syndrome) (see Chapter 3, III, F)
        d. Palatal myoclonus (see Chapter 3, III, J)

BIBLIOGRAPHY

Books

Jankovic J, Tolosa E, eds. *Advances in Neurology. Facial Dyskinesias.* Vol 49. New York, NY: Raven Press; 1988.

Chapters

Burde RM, Savino PJ, Trobe JD. *Clinical Decisions in Neuro-Ophthalmology.* 3rd ed. St Louis, Mo: CV Mosby; 2002:276-296.

Landa M, Bedrossian EH. Blepharoptosis. In: Della Rocca RC, Bedrossian EH, Arthurs BP. *Ophthalmic Plastic Surgery: Decision Making and Techniques.* New York, NY: McGraw-Hill; 2002:77-89.

McCord CD, Tanenbaum M, Nunnery W, eds. *Oculoplastic Surgery.* 3rd ed. New York, NY: Raven Press; 1995:329-375.

Skarf B. Normal and abnormal eyelid function. In: Miller NR, Newman NJ, eds. *Walsh and Hoyt's Clinical Neuro-Ophthalmology.* 6th ed. Vol 1. Philadelphia, Pa: Lippincott Williams & Wilkins; 2005:1177-1229.

Articles

Boghen D. Apraxia of lid opening: a review. *Neurology.* 1997;48:1491-1494.

Cogan DG. Myasthenia gravis: a review of the disease and a description of lid twitch as a characteristic sign. *Arch Ophthalmol.* 1965;74:217-221.

Hallett M. Blepharospasm: recent advances. *Neurology.* 2002;59:1306-1312.

Janetta PJ, Abbasy M, Maroon JC, et al. Etiology and definitive microsurgical treatment of hemifacial spasm: operative techniques and results in 47 patients. *J Neurosurg*. 1977;47:321.

Schmidtke K, Buttner-Ennever JA. Nervous control of eyelid function: a review of clinical, experimental and pathological data. *Brain*. 1992;115:227-247.

Chapter 15

Headache

John E. Carter, MD

I. **Classification of headache: the International Headache Society (IHS)**

    A.   The IHS divides headache into 13 classifications (Table 15-1)

    B.   Headache may be broadly divided into the primary headache syndromes such as migraine and the secondary headaches due to an underlying disorder such as giant cell arteritis, idiopathic intracranial hypertension, or brain tumor

    C.   Primary headache disorders account for 90% of patients presenting with headache

    D.   This chapter will concentrate on the primary and secondary headache syndromes with important neuro-ophthalmologic manifestations or implications

II. **Migraine**

    A.   Paroxysmal disorder affecting approximately 15% of women and 5% of men in the United States

    B.   This compares to tension-type headache (muscle contraction headache) that affects about 80% of the population

    C.   Phases of migraine. Migraine attacks have several phases and most patients experience more than one phase

        1.   Prodrome: premonitory symptoms occur hours to days before the onset of headache in 60% of patients

            a.   Psychological: depression, euphoria, irritability, restlessness and hyperactivity, drowsiness, mental fatigue, and mental slowness

            b.   Neurologic: photophobia, phonophobia, hyperosmia

            c.   Constitutional: sluggishness, increased thirst and urination, fluid retention, food cravings, anorexia, diarrhea, or constipation

        2.   Aura

            a.   Focal neurologic symptoms preceding or accompanying or rarely occurring after an attack of migraine

            b.   Experienced by 20% of migraineurs

            c.   Most develop in a progressive fashion over 5 to 20 minutes and last less than 60 minutes

Table 15-1

ABBREVIATED CLASSIFICATION OF HEADACHE

1.   Migraine
     1.1   Migraine without aura
     1.2   Migraine with aura including typical aura without headache, familial hemiplegic migraine, and basilar-type migraine
     1.3   Childhood periodic syndromes that may be precursors to or associated with migraine
     1.4   Retinal migraine
     1.5   Complications of migraine
          1.5.1   Chronic migraine
          1.5.2   Status migrainosus
          1.5.3   Persistent aura without infarction
2.   Tension-type headache
3.   Cluster headache and other trigeminal autonomic cephalalgias
     3.1   Cluster headache
     3.2   Paroxysmal hemicrania
     3.3   SUNCT—short-lasting unilateral neuralgiform headache attacks with conjunctival injection and tearing
4.   Other primary headaches including cough headache, exertional headache, headache associated with sexual activity
5.   Headache associated with head and/or neck trauma
6.   Headache associated with vascular disorders
     6.1   Headache associated with stroke
     6.2   Unruptured vascular malformation including aneurysm, arteriovenous malformation, dural arteriovenous fistula
     6.3   Arteritis including giant cell arteritis
     6.4   Arterial dissection
     6.5   Cerebral venous thrombosis
     6.6   CADASIL—cerebral autosomal dominant arteriopathy with subcortical infarcts and leukoencephalopathy
     6.7   MELAS—mitochondrial encephalopathy, lactic acidosis, and stroke-like episodes
     6.8   Pituitary apoplexy
7.   Headache associated with nonvascular intracranial disorders
     7.1   High CSF pressure
     7.2   Low CSF pressure
     7.3   Noninfectious inflammatory disease
     7.4   Intracranial neoplasm
8.   Headache associated with drugs or their withdrawal
9.   Headache attributed to infection
10. Headache attributed to disorder of homeostasis hypoxia/hypercapnea including high-altitude headache, diving headache, and sleep apnea headache; hypertension
11. Headache or facial pain associated with disorder of cranium, neck, eyes, ears, nose, sinuses, teeth, mouth, or other facial or cranial structures

continued on next page

Table 15-1 (continued)

ABBREVIATED CLASSIFICATION OF HEADACHE

12. Headache attributed to psychiatric disorder
13. Cranial neuralgias, nerve trunk pain, and deafferentation pain
    - 13.1 Trigeminal neuralgia
    - 13.2 Glossopharyngeal neuralgia
    - 13.3 Nervus intermedius neuralgia
    - 13.4 Occipital neuralgia
    - 13.5 Cold-stimulus headache
    - 13.6 Head or face pain due to Herpes zoster
    - 13.7 Tolosa-Hunt syndrome
    - 13.8 Ophthalmoplegic "migraine"

Modified from the International Headache Society Classification of Headache.

      d. Most frequently aura consists of visual symptoms but sensory, motor, language, and brainstem symptoms may occur

      e. Visual aura: bright, angular, positive visual sensations often described as sparkles, flashes of color, or heat waves (Figure 15-1). Usually of a hemianopic nature, lasts less than 1 hour, with typical "buildup" and "march"

      f. Occasional patients experience aura without headache (acephalgic migraine)

   3. Headache phase

      a. Headache is usually unilateral at onset and is characterized as throbbing

      b. Headache often becomes pancephalgic and the throbbing changes to a steady, aching pain

      c. Nausea almost always accompanies migraine without aura

      d. Vomiting may occur at the height of the attack and signal the end of the headache phase or may begin an intensifying phase of the headache

      e. Photophobia and phonophobia accompany the headache in most patients

      f. Ocular symptoms and signs include conjunctival injection, periorbital swelling, and excessive tearing

      g. Headache usually lasts from 4 to 24 hours. Headache lasting longer than 72 hours is called status migrainosus

   4. Postdromal phase

      a. In some patients, especially migraine with aura, the headache resolves with a period of sleep

      b. After the headache the patient is often left with malaise for 24 to 48 hours

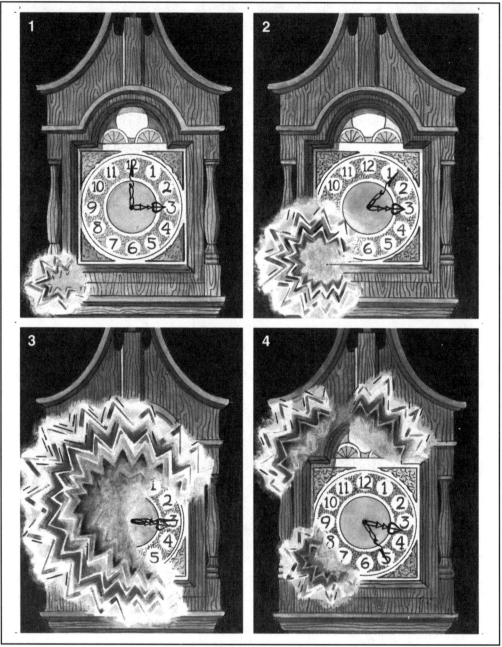

Figure 15-1. Scintillating fortification scotoma of migraine appears in one portion of the visual field, typically enlarges to cover central fixation, then "marches" toward the periphery and breaks apart. The entire phenomenon lasts 15 to 30 minutes. (Reprinted with permission from Hupp SL, Kline LB, Corbett JJ. Visual disturbances of migraine. *Surv Ophthalmol.* 1989;33:221-236.) **Please see the four-color tearout page at the back of the book.**

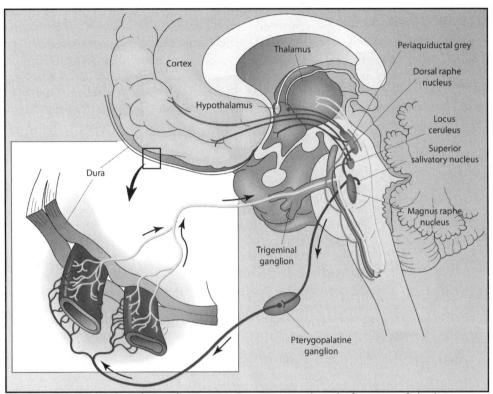

Figure 15-2. Pathophysiology of migraine. Migraine involves dysfunction of the brainstem pathways that normally modulate sensory input. Trigeminovascular input from the meningeal vessels passes through the trigeminal ganglion and synapses on second-order neurons in the trigeminocervical complex. These second-order neurons project to the thalamus. This trigeminal-autonomic reflex is present in normal persons and is expressed most strongly in patients with trigeminal-autonomic cephalgias, such as cluster headache and paroxysmal hemicrania; it may be active in migraine. Brain imaging studies suggest that important modulation of the trigeminovascular nociceptive input comes from the dorsal raphe nucleus, locus ceruleus, and nucleus raphe magnus in the brainstem. (From *Headache in Clinical Practice*. 2nd ed, Silberstein SD, Lipton RB, Goadsby PJ, © 2002 Martin Dunitz. Reproduced by permission of Taylor & Francis Books UK.)

D. Pathophysiology of migraine: the trigeminovascular system and the neural hypothesis of migraine (Figure 15-2)

1. The possible mechanisms of pain in migraine involves the cranial blood vessels, changes in the dura mater, and changes in the modulation of nociceptive input to the central nervous system

2. The vessels and the dura mater of the anterior and middle cranial fossa are innervated by the ophthalmic division of the trigeminal nerve. The dura of the posterior fossa is innervated by the branches of C2

3. Stimulation of cranial vascular afferents activates neurons in the trigeminal nucleus within the brainstem and the dorsal horns at C1 and C2 (trigeminocervical complex)

4. Second-order neurons in the trigeminocervical complex project through the brainstem and to the thalamus

5.   A reflex connection in the superior salivatory nucleus in the pons produces cranial parasympathetic outflow to the dura and cranial vessels via the ptery-gopalatine, otic and carotid ganglia, termed the trigeminoautonomic reflex

6.   An axon reflex produces local release of neuropeptides from trigeminal sensory axons onto cranial arteries, meningeal tissues, dural arteries, and dural sinuses, promoting local vasodilation and plasma extravasation. Referred to as neurogenic inflammation, this sets up a pain-sensitive state. Throbbing pain may be the result of normal pulsations of cranial blood vessels or normal pulsations of cerebrospinal fluid (CSF)

7.   Serotonin (5-hydroxytriptamine or 5HT) is a key neurotransmitter in migraine

   a.   5HT receptors on cranial vessels have a vasoconstrictive action

   b.   5HT receptors on the terminals of trigeminal nerve axons have an inhibitory action

   c.   Drugs specifically effective in aborting migraine attacks, both ergots and triptans, are 5HT receptor agonists. Some prophylactic drugs useful in migraine are serotonergic

8.   Although controversial, there is increasing evidence for an increased state of excitability in the brains of migraineurs, not just during attacks but between attacks. This may be related to dysfunction in the serotonergic dorsal raphe nuclei of the brainstem

E.   Migraine without aura (common migraine)

   1.   Diagnostic criteria are shown in Table 15-2

F.   Migraine with aura (classic migraine)

   1.   Diagnostic criteria are shown in Table 15-3

   2.   The features of migrainous visual aura are so characteristic as to be diagnostic

   3.   Note that a diagnosis of migraine with aura can be made without the presence of headache even though that is uncommon

   4.   Pearl: remember that over a lifetime a given patient may start with migraine with aura and later evolve to a pattern of migraine without aura or vice versa

G.   Retinal (ocular) migraine is an uncommon form of migraine consisting of repeated attacks of monocular visual loss lasting less than 1 hour and associated with headache

   1.   Many patients experiencing homonymous visual field defects attribute the defect to the eye on the involved side. Confirmation of the monocular nature requires an observant patient testing each eye individually to confirm that the visual loss is limited to a single eye

   2.   IHS criteria are at least two attacks of fully reversible monocular visual loss lasting less than 60 minutes followed by a headache within 60 minutes but sometimes preceding the visual loss

   3.   Typically patients are young (<50 years) and already have a history of migraine with or without aura

   4.   Patients with migraine and monocular visual loss have been described with arterial and venous retinal vascular occlusion, central serous retinopathy, vitreous hemorrhage, retinal hemorrhage, and anterior and posterior ischemic optic neuropathy

---

Table 15-2

DIAGNOSTIC CRITERIA FOR MIGRAINE WITHOUT AURA

A.   Headache lasts 4 to 72 hours
B.   Headache has at least two of the following characteristics:
   1.   Unilateral location
   2.   Pulsating quality
   3.   Moderate or severe intensity inhibiting daily activities
   4.   Aggravation by routine physical activity
C.   At least one of the following occurs during headache:
   1.   Nausea and/or vomiting
   2.   Photophobia and phonophobia

Table 15-3

DIAGNOSTIC CRITERIA FOR MIGRAINE WITH AURA

A.   At least three of the following four characteristics are present:
   1.   One or more fully reversible aura symptoms indicate focal cerebral cortical or brain-stem dysfunction
   2.   At least one aura symptom develops gradually over more than 4 minutes or two or more symptoms occur in succession
   3.   No single aura symptom lasts more than 60 minutes
   4.   Headache follows aura within 60 minutes or begins before or simultaneously with the aura
B.   Headache has at least two of the following characteristics:
   1.   Unilateral location
   2.   Pulsating quality
   3.   Moderate or severe intensity inhibiting daily activities
   4.   Aggravation by routine physical activity
C.   At least one of the following occurs during headache:
   1.   Nausea and/or vomiting
   2.   Photophobia and phonophobia

---

     5.   More recently it has been suggested the term "retinal migraine" be replaced with more general designation of "retinal vasospasm"
     6.   Because it is uncommon and because other conditions may mimic it, retinal migraine is a diagnosis of exclusion
     7.   Treatment:
        a.   Calcium channel blockers
        b.   Beta-blockers
  H.   "Basilar-type" migraine

   1. Initially proposed by Bickerstaff and formerly referred to as basilar artery migraine, the new IHS classification considers migraine patients with aura symptoms attributable to brainstem or cerebellar dysfunction as being another variant of migraine with aura
   2. Neurologic symptoms include ataxia, diplopia, dysarthria, vertigo, tinnitus, facial or limb paresthesias, and disturbance of vision
   3. Visual symptoms are bilateral and may include:
       a. Dimming or total loss of sight
       b. Visual hallucinations or unformed images
       c. Photopsias

I. Complications of migraine
   1. Migrainous stroke
       a. Patients may have migraine and stroke coincidentally
       b. Occasionally patients with stroke experience migrainous symptoms such as positive neurologic symptoms or a buildup of the neurologic deficits, a migraine mimic. When occurring in an older patient who has continued to suffer from migraine it may be difficult to distinguish from other forms of stroke and requires a workup directed at causes of stroke
       c. When a migraineur has a typical aura during the course of a typical migraine but the neurologic deficit persists then the stroke may be attributed to the migraine. However, other causes of stroke still must be excluded by diagnostic studies
       d. It has been hypothesized that migraine-induced neurologic deficits are not the result of ischemia but of excitotoxicity caused by dysfunction of serotonergic pathways and fatal "neuronal overdrive" resulting in cell death with free radical formation and nitric oxide effects
       e. In young cohorts (<50 years) with stroke, 10% to 15% of patients have migraine; a majority of these are women who are also on oral contraceptives. Young women with migraine have a stroke-risk several times their peers and this risk is magnified by use of tobacco and oral contraceptives
   2. Persistent aura in migraine
       a. Rarely, patients with migraine experience positive visual symptoms during periods between migraine attacks. Besides supporting the concept of neuronal hyperexcitability in migraine, it is important to recognize these are related to migraine and reassure the patients of their benign nature

J. Treatment of migraine
   1. Nonpharmacologic therapy
       a. Lifestyle changes: regular sleep, regular meals, exercise
       b. Dietary triggers may include alcohol, red wine, certain cheeses, and other foodstuffs
   2. Abortive therapy to treat the individual headaches are of two types
       a. Nonspecific treatments such as aspirin, acetaminophen, nonsteroidal anti-inflammatory drugs, opiates, and combination analgesics
       b. Migraine-specific treatments
           i. Ergot derivatives (ergotamine, caffergot, dihydroergotamine [DHE])

        ii.   Triptans (sumatriptan, rizatriptan, zolmitriptan, naratriptan, eletriptan, almotriptan)

    3.   Preventive therapy is indicated in patients experiencing more frequent attacks and should be considered in patients experiencing headache 1 or more days per week. A wide variety of drugs are used as prophylactic therapy, only some of which have been demonstrated effective in controlled clinical trials

        a.   Beta-blockers (propranolol, metoprolol)

        b.   Calcium-channel blockers (verapamil)

        c.   Tricyclic antidepressants (amitriptyline, nortriptyline)

        d.   Serotonin reuptake inhibitors (fluoxetine, paroxetine, sertraline)

        e.   Trazodone

        f.   Anticonvulsants: valproic acid, topiramate, gabapentin

III.   Tension-type headache (muscle contraction headache)

    A.   Typical symptoms include bilateral headache, often with posterior neck tightness. The headache is dull and may be likened to pressure or a band-like or vise-like sensation

    B.   Exercise does not worsen the pain and may relieve it

    C.   Nausea and vomiting, photophobia, phonophobia are not features of tension-type headache

    D.   As migraine may be associated with psychologic stress, occurring during or sometimes after relief of the stressful situation, so tension-type headache may occur during identifiable psychologic stress

    E.   There is substantial overlap in the actual pain experience of patients with migraine and tension-type headache:

        1.   Tension-type headache may start or be worse on one side

        2.   One third of patients with migraine without aura have bilateral headache from the outset and many more have unilateral headache initially which subsequently generalizes

        3.   The occiput and posterior neck is a common site of pain in both groups

IV.   Cluster and other trigeminal autonomic cephalgias

    A.   Diagnostic criteria for cluster headache are listed in Table 15-4

    B.   Cluster headache is the most common trigeminal autonomic cephalgia

    C.   Typically characterized by unilateral attacks of short-lived (<60 minutes) but very severe pain associated with rhinorrhea, lacrimation, and Horner's syndrome

    D.   Attacks may occur one or more times daily, often in the early morning and repeating the same pattern each day

    E.   In distinction to migraine, most patients with cluster become restless and move around during the attack

    F.   Clusters may last from weeks to months and may be seasonal

    G.   Individual headaches may be treated with oxygen, parenteral triptans, or DHE

    H.   Cluster periods are managed with corticosteroids, daily triptan administration, and methysergide. Verapamil and lithium have been used successfully as well

    I.   SUNCT—short-lasting unilateral neuralgiform headache attacks with conjunctival injection and tearing is a newly recognized trigeminal autonomic cephalgia

Table 15-4

DIAGNOSTIC CRITERIA FOR CLUSTER HEADACHE

A. Severe unilateral orbital, supraorbital, and/or temporal pain lasts 15 to 180 minutes untreated

B. Headache is associated with at least one of the following on the side of the pain:
1. Conjunctival injection
2. Lacrimation
3. Nasal congestion
4. Rhinorrhea
5. Forehead and facial sweating
6. Miosis
7. Ptosis
8. Eyelid edema

C. Frequency of attacks ranges from one every other day to eight per day

---

1. Projectile lacrimation may occur
2. Episodes usually last 5 seconds to 5 minutes but usually occur 25 times a day
3. Magnetic resonance imaging (MRI) is necessary to exclude a secondary cause including pituitary adenoma and posterior fossa tumors, demyelinating disease, and vascular compression of the trigeminal nerve
4. Best treatment: anticonvulsants (topiramate, lamotrigine), carbamazepine. SUNCT often worsens with corticosteroids and calcium channel blockers

V. Secondary headache syndromes

A. Some secondary headaches have important neuro-ophthalmologic implications. Systemic symptoms and signs and past medical history are critical in directing laboratory evaluations in these cases

B. Giant cell arteritis
1. New onset of headache in patient over 50 years
2. Bitemporal
3. Scalp tenderness
4. Jaw claudication
5. Polymyalgia
6. Visual symptoms (see Chapter 9)

C. Carotid or vertebral arterial dissection
1. Ophthalmic manifestations: carotid dissection produces an ipsilateral Horner's syndrome and may be associated with retinal or optic nerve ischemia and occasionally ocular motor cranial nerve palsies and hemispheric stroke. Vertebral artery dissection produces brainstem stroke
2. Associated symptoms and signs: ipsilateral neck or head pain with or without contralateral hemiparesis; dysgeusia

3. Diagnostic evaluation should include MRI, magnetic resonance angiography (MRA), computed tomographic angiography (CTA), and possibly cerebral angiography

4. Treatment: antiplatelet therapy, anticoagulation, carotid stenting

D. Cerebral venous thrombosis

1. Ophthalmic manifestations: papilledema, VI nerve palsy

2. Associated symptoms and signs: seizures, contralateral hemiparesis, obtundation

3. Diagnostic evaluation should include MRI, magnetic resonance venography (MRV)

E. Pituitary apoplexy

1. Pituitary adenoma may outgrow its blood supply and experience spontaneous hemorrhagic necrosis. Sudden increase in size of the mass compresses the optic chiasm and extension into the cavernous sinuses damages the ocular motor cranial nerves

2. Ophthalmic manifestations: acute ophthalmoparesis, acute visual loss

3. Associated symptoms and signs include severe headache, photophobia, meningismus

4. Diagnostic evaluation should include MRI. Hemorrhage or cystic change is seen within pituitary mass

5. Treatment consists endocrinologic support and possible pituitary surgery

F. Intracranial hypertension, papilledema, and idiopathic intracranial hypertension

1. Increased intracranial pressure may be due to obstructive hydrocephalus, a space-occupying lesion, arteriovenous malformation, dural arteriovenous fistula, or meningeal processes including infection and non-infectious inflammation. In the absence of one of these processes, the correct diagnosis is idiopathic intracranial hypertension or pseudotumor cerebri (see Chapter 9, IV)

2. Headache of increased intracranial pressure:
   a. Usually appears quite suddenly
   b. May be mild or intermittent initially, but progressively worsens
   c. May be worse in head-down position, coughing, straining

G. Intracranial hypotension

1. Commonly seen after lumbar puncture; patients experience headache present when upright and resolves when lying down

2. Syndrome of spontaneous intracranial hypotension is recognized by this same posture-dependent headache

3. MRI findings include:
   a. Diffuse enhancement of the dura
   b. Sagging of the brain with descent of the cerebellar tonsils into the foramen magnum
   c. Decreased size of the CSF cisterns
   d. Pituitary gland may be enlarged and the chiasm draped over it
   e. Subdural fluid collections may develop

       4.   On lumbar puncture, opening pressure may be normal but is usually low or unmeasurable

H.   Microvascular ocular motor cranial nerve infarcts
       1.   Ophthalmic manifestations: III (pupil-sparing), IV, or VI nerve palsy usually in setting of diabetes mellitus or hypertension
       2.   Associated symptoms and signs include pain around the eye, possibly due to meningeal ischemia, which may precede the diplopia by up to a week
       3.   Pain resolves within 1 to 2 weeks
       4.   Severity of the pain is not a distinctive feature when comparing microvascular and aneurysmal III nerve palsy

I.   Ophthalmoplegic migraine (see Chapter 5)
       1.   Diagnostic criteria: at least two attacks of a migraine-like headache accompanied or followed within 4 days of onset by paresis of one or more of III, IV, or VI cranial nerves and not attributable to parasellar, superior orbital fissure or posterior fossa lesions
       2.   Onset usually before age 10; on occasion begins in adulthood
       3.   III nerve affected 10 to 1 over VI nerve
       4.   Pupil and accommodation frequently involved
       5.   Ophthalmoplegia occurs at height of headache, persisting when headache clears (may last days to weeks)
       6.   Strict criteria for diagnosis
           a.   Onset usually in first decade of life
           b.   History of typical migraine
           c.   Ophthalmoplegia ipsilateral to headache
           d.   MR scanning: normal or enhancement of involved ocular motor cranial nerve
       7.   MRI findings suggest condition may be due to structural lesion (schwannoma, angioma), ischemia, or demyelination at the nerve exit zone

J.   Herpes zoster ophthalmicus
       1.   Ophthalmic manifestations:
           a.   Keratitis
           b.   Uveitis
           c.   Ophthalmoplegia due to vasculitis of vasa nervorum of ocular motor cranial nerves or orbital myositis
           d.   Optic neuritis—papillitis or retrobulbar
           e.   Vasculitis involving cranial arteries may produce homonymous hemianopia due to stroke
       2.   Associated symptoms and signs: pain followed within days by vesicular eruption in the distribution of the ophthalmic division of the trigeminal nerve
       3.   Acute treatment
           a.   Corticosteroid
           b.   Antiviral—acyclovir, famvir
       4.   Post-herpetic neuralgia
           a.   Carbamazepine
           b.   Gabapentin

Table 15-5

RED FLAGS IN PATIENTS WITH HEADACHE

Sudden onset headache	Subarachnoid hemorrhage, bleeding into arteriovenous malformation (AVM) or neoplasm, posterior fossa mass with developing hydrocephalus
Progressive headache	Mass lesion, subdural hematoma, medication overuse
Systemic symptoms accompanying headache (fever, rash, neck stiffness, jaw or tongue pain)	Giant cell or other arteritis, meningitis, encephalitis, Lyme disease, systemic infection, collagen vascular disease
Focal neurologic symptoms other than typical visual or sensory aura of migraine or persistent focal neurologic symptoms or signs	AVM, mass lesion, collagen vascular disease, stroke
Papilledema	Intracranial mass or hemorrhage, encephalitis or meningitis, idiopathic intracranial hypertension
Triggered by cough, exertion, valsalva maneuver, or head or neck movements	Carotid or vertebral dissection, subarachnoid hemorrhage, mass lesion
Headache during pregnancy or peripartum period	Idiopathic intracranial hypertension, cortical vein or cranial venous sinus thrombosis, carotid dissection, pituitary apoplexy
New headache in patients with:	
Cancer	Metastases
HIV	Opportunistic infection, lymphoma
Lyme disease	Meningoencephalitis

VI. **Table 15-5 emphasizes worrisome signs or symptoms accompanying headache and important considerations in differential diagnosis**

BIBLIOGRAPHY

Books

Oleson J, Tfelt-Hansen P, Welch KMA, et al. *The Headaches.* 3rd ed. Philadelphia, Pa: Lippincott Williams & Wilkins; 2006.

Silberstein SD, Lipton RB, Goadsby PJ. *Headache in Clinical Practice.* London: Martin Dunitz Ltd; 2002.

Chapters

Troost BT. Migraine and other headaches. In: Glaser JS, ed. *Neuro-Ophthalmology*. 3rd ed. Philadelphia, Pa: Lippincott Williams & Wilkins; 1999:553-587.

Van Stavern GP. Headache and facial pain. In: Miller NR, Newman NJ, eds. *Walsh and Hoyt's Clinical Neuro-Ophthalmology*. 6th ed. Vol 1. Philadelphia, Pa: Lippincott Williams & Wilkins; 2005:1275-1311.

Articles

Bousser MG. Estrogens, migraine, tobacco, and stroke. *Stroke*. 2004;35(Suppl 1):2652-2656.

Eggers AE. New neural theory of migraine. *Med Hypotheses*. 2001;56:360-363.

Goadsby PJ. The pharmacology of headache. *Prog Neurobiol*. 2000;62:509-525.

Goadsby PJ, Lipton RB, Ferrari MD. Drug therapy: migraine—current understanding and treatment. *N Engl J Med*. 2002;346:257-270.

Headache Classification Subcommittee of the International Headache Society. The International Classification of Headache Disorders. 2nd ed. *Cephalalgia*. 2004;24(Suppl 1).

Lipton RB, Silberstein SD, Saper JR, Bigal ME, Goadsby PJ. Why headache treatment fails. *Neurology*. 2003;70:1064-1070.

Liu GT, Schatz NJ, Galetta SL, Volpe NJ, Skobieranda F, Kosmorsky GS. Persistent positive visual phenomena in migraine. *Neurology*. 1995;45:664-668.

Mark AS, Blake PA, Atlas SW, et al. Gd-DPTA enhancement of the cisternal portion of the oculomotor nerve on MR imaging. *AJNR*. 1992;13:1463-1470.

May A, Goadsby PJ. Pharmacological opportunities and pitfalls in the therapy of migraine. *Curr Opin Neurol*. 2001;14:341-345.

Welch KMA. Pathogenesis of migraine. *Sem Neurol*. 1997;17:335-341.

Winterkorn JM, Kupersmith MJ, Wirtschafter JD, Forman S. Treatment of vasospastic amaurosis fugax with calcium-channel blockers. *N Engl J Med*. 1993;329:396-398.

Chapter 16

Carotid Artery Disease and the Eye

Milton F. White, Jr, MD

I. **General considerations**

   A. Carotid artery arteriosclerosis accounts for 20% to 50% of all strokes

   B. Cerebrovascular insufficiency is often accompanied by ocular signs and symptoms

   C. Depending upon the clinical setting, there is a spectrum of stroke risk (Table 16-1)

II. **Anatomy of the carotid system**

   A. The first major branch of the aortic arch is the innominate artery, which gives rise to the right common carotid artery

   B. The left common carotid is the second major branch of the aortic arch

   C. Each common carotid artery divides into internal and external branches at the C4 level, about 3 cm below the angle of the mandible

   D. The internal carotid artery enters the skull through the carotid canal of the temporal bone, ascends along the side of the sella turcica, forms the carotid siphon as it passes through the cavernous sinus, then emerges intracranially

   E   The ophthalmic artery is its first major branch, and the internal carotid ultimately divides into the anterior and middle cerebral arteries

   F. Numerous connections between the external and internal carotid systems involve the ophthalmic artery (Figure 16-1)

   G. Third-order neuron (postganglionic) sympathetic fibers to eye, orbit, and face travel in the posterior carotid sheath

   H. Cervical portion of carotid artery is surgically accessible

III. **Ocular manifestations of carotid disease**

   A. Transient monocular visual loss (TMVL)

   1. Alternate terms: amaurosis fugax ("fleeting blindness"), transient monocular blindness

   2. Duration: 2 to 30 minutes

Table 16-1

SPECTRUM OF STROKE RISK

Patient Group	Risk of Stroke Per Year (%)
No carotid disease	0.1
Asymptomatic carotid bruit	0.1 to 0.4
Transient monocular visual loss	2.0
Asymptomatic carotid stenosis	2.5
Retinal infarcts, emboli	3.0
Transient cerebral ischemic attack	8.0

Modified from Trobe JD. Carotid endarterectomy: who needs it? *Ophthalmology.* 1987;94:725-730.

3. Typically, a "shade" temporarily covers part or all of visual field. Other descriptions include a "dark cloud," "a film," or generalized darkening

4. Visual loss may include entire visual field or only half or a quadrant of the field

5. Positive visual phenomena may be described by one-third of patients

6. TMVL associated with carotid stenosis is most commonly due to embolic disease (see below)

7. Less common pathophysiologic mechanisms include diminished blood flow (hypoperfusion) and vasospasm of the ophthalmic and/or central retinal artery

8. Occasionally, amaurosis fugax can be precipitated by exposure to bright light (photostress: retinal vascular insufficiency to photoreceptors)

9. Natural history of TMVL:
    a. Risk of permanent visual loss—1% per year
    b. Risk of stroke—2% per year (20 times higher than patient without carotid disease) (see Table 16-1)
    c. Mortality rate—2% to 4% per year
    d. Main cause of death—cardiac disease
    e. TMVL with associated visible retinal emboli—mortality rate increases to 4% to 6% per year
    f. No relationship between frequency or duration of visual symptoms and risk of stroke

10. A variety of other conditions cause TMVL (Table 16-2)

B. Retinal circulatory emboli
    1. Platelet-fibrin
        a. Fisher plugs
        b. White intra-arterial plugs lodge at bifurcations
        c. Source: internal carotid artery atheroma and ulceration
    2. Cholesterol
        a. Hollenhorst plaques

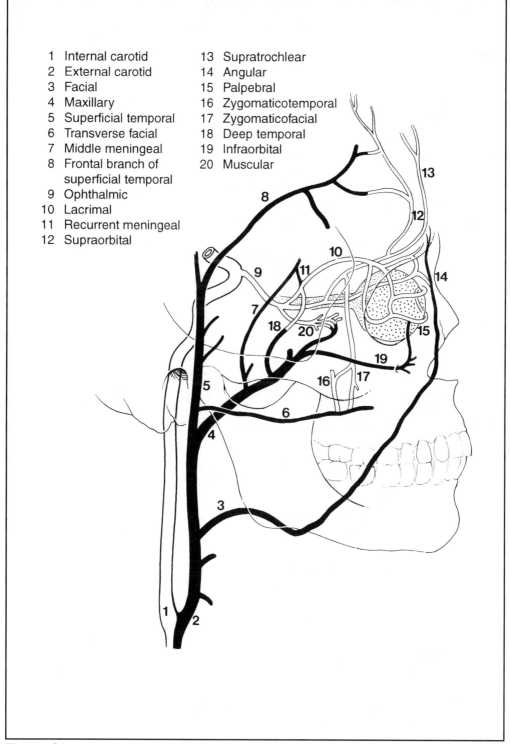

1 Internal carotid
2 External carotid
3 Facial
4 Maxillary
5 Superficial temporal
6 Transverse facial
7 Middle meningeal
8 Frontal branch of
   superficial temporal
9 Ophthalmic
10 Lacrimal
11 Recurrent meningeal
12 Supraorbital
13 Supratrochlear
14 Angular
15 Palpebral
16 Zygomaticotemporal
17 Zygomaticofacial
18 Deep temporal
19 Infraorbital
20 Muscular

Figure 16-1. Anastomotic connection between the internal and external carotid arteries. Note the key position of the ophthalmic artery (9).

Table 16-2

CONDITIONS ASSOCIATED WITH TRANSIENT MONOCULAR VISUAL LOSS

Intraocular	**Carotid Artery**	**Other Conditions**
Tear film abnormalities	Embolism	Hypertension
Hyphema	Thrombosis	Hypotension
UGH syndrome	Dissection	Hyperglycemia
Impending CRVO		Migraine
Vitreous debris	**Cardiac**	Raynaud's phenomenon
Glaucoma	Embolism	Antiphospholipid antibodies
Papilledema	Arrhythmia	Non-organic visual loss
Disc drusen	Valvular disease	
Congenital anomalies of the optic disc		
Ischemic optic neuropathy	**Hematologic**	
	Anemia	
Intraorbital	Polycythemia	
Hemangioma	Sickle cell disease	
Osteoma	Thrombocytosis	

Intracranial
Ateriovenous malformation
Tumor

Modified from Seybold ME. Nonembolic sources of amaurosis fugax. In: Bernstein EF, ed. *Amaurosis Fugax.* New York, NY: Springer-Verlag; 1988:168-173.

      b.   Bright, orange-yellow, refractile

      c.   Source: carotid and aortic atheroma

   3.   Calcium

      a.   Gray-white, nonrefractile

      b.   Usually lodge in retinal arterioles near or on the optic disc

      c.   Source: cardiac valves or aortic wall

   4.   Septic vegetation—bacterial endocarditis

   5.   Fat—due to long bone fracture

   6.   Myxoma—heart

   7.   Amniotic fluid—uterus

   8.   Rare—mercury, air, paraffin

 C.   Retinal arterial occlusion

   1.   Types:

      a.   Central retinal artery occlusion (CRAO)

      b.   Branch retinal artery occlusion (BRAO)

   2.   Central retinal artery has narrowest diameter at lamina cribrosa, where it is most vulnerable to occlusion

3. Five major causes of CRAO:
   a. Embolization
   b. Localized atheromatous stenosis
   c. Arteritic obliteration
   d. Reduced vascular perfusion
   e. Vasospasm
4. Patient with CRAO reports painless loss of vision
5. CRAO persisting greater than 100 minutes leads to permanent loss of vision
6. Clinical findings with CRAO
   a. Segmentation of blood in retinal arterioles—"box-carring"
   b. Visible emboli in 11% to 20% of patients
   c. Axoplasmic flow stasis with retinal edema or "whitening"
   d. "Cherry-red" macular spot
   e. After several days retinal swelling subsides; loss of retinal nerve fiber layer (NFL); optic atrophy (4 to 8 weeks)
   f. Arteries may demonstrate both narrowing and sheathing
7. Clinical findings in BRAO
   a. Segmentation of blood in involved branch retinal arteriole—"box-carring"
   b. Visible emboli in 60% to 68% of patients
   c. Retinal edema localized to area of involved arteriole
   d. With resolution of retinal swelling, area of NFL atrophy; segmental optic atrophy
8. Emergency treatment of CRAO
   a. Immediate goal is to increase perfusion and preserve flow in the CRAO:
      i. Lower intraocular pressure
      ii. Vasodilation
   b. Lower intraocular pressure: anterior chamber paracentesis, ocular massage, topical beta-blocker, topical carbonic anhydrase inhibitor
   c. Vasodilation: breathe into paper bag, inhalation of carbogen (95% O_2, 5% CO_2), intravenous aminophylline, retrobulbar anesthesia
   d. All treatment modalities are empiric; none proven due to lack of controlled studies
9. Survival time of 5.5 years following CRAO vs expected survival of 15 years in age-matched population
10. Three to 10% of patients older than 50 years with CRAO have giant cell arteritis. Remember to obtain a Westergren sedimentation rate STAT!

D. Evaluation and therapy for patients with amaurosis fugax and retinal arterial occlusions
   1. Careful history searching for vascular risk factors:
      a. Hypertension
      b. Diabetes mellitus
      c. Hypercholesterolemia/hyperlipidemia
      d. Tobacco use

Table 16-3

EVALUATION OF THE PATIENT WITH OCULAR ISCHEMIA

History

Physical Examination
Eye
Neck (extracranial carotid artery)
Heart

Hematologic
CBC, platelet count, ESR, PT, PTT
Chemistry profile, serum lipids
ANA, FTA-Abs

Diagnostic Procedures
Chest radiology
EKG
Carotid duplex scanning
Magnetic resonance angiography
Selected patients:
Echocardiography
Carotid angiography

Selected patients:

Hypercoagulable states (protein C, S deficiency; Factor V Leiden deficiency; antithrombin III; antiphospholipid antibodies; G20210A mutation; homocysteinemia)

Hyperviscosity syndromes (polycythemia; sickle cell disease; thrombocytosis)

Modified from Carter JE. Carotid artery disease and its ocular manifestations. *Ophthalmol Clin North Am.* 1992;5:425-443.

e.   Cardiac disease: ischemic, valvular, arrhythmia

2.   Diagnostic studies are summarized in Table 16-3

3.   Treatment

   a.   Medical

      i.   Reduction of vascular risk factors

      ii.   Aspirin

      iii. Dipyridamole-aspirin (Aggrenox [Boehringer Ingelheim Pharmaceuticals, Ingelheim, Germany])

      iv.   Clopidogrel (Plavix [Bristol-Myers Squibb, New York, NY])

      v.   Coumadin (Bristol-Myers Squibb)

   b.   Surgical

      i.   Cardiac—if source of emboli

      ii.   Carotid—North American Symptomatic Carotid Endarterectomy Trial (NASCET): endarterectomy recommended for all patients with symptomatic extracranial stenosis of 70% or greater whose medical condition does not preclude surgery (Table 16-4)

      iii. **Remember:** consider the surgical perioperative morbidity/mortality rate of your patient vs the natural history of the disease (see Table 16-1) when considering surgical intervention

      iv.   More recent NASCET data found, in patients with TMVL, six factors increased stroke risk:

         a.   Age >75 years

Table 16-4

HIGH-RISK FACTORS FOR CAROTID ENDARTERECTOMY PERIOPERATIVE STROKE/DEATH

Age ≥70 years
Refractory hypertension
Severe coronary disease
Severe obstructive pulmonary disease
Marked obesity
Recent or multiple strokes
Bilateral carotid stenosis
Distal ipsilateral carotid stenosis

Modified from Carter JE. Carotid artery disease and its ocular manifestations. *Ophthalmol Clin North Am.* 1992;5:425-443.

Table 16-5

IMPACT OF RISK FACTORS ON TRANSIENT MONOCULAR VISUAL LOSS
3-YEAR RISK OF IPSILATERAL STROKE

Risk Factors	Medical (%)	Surgical (%)	Stroke Risk Reduction (medical minus surgical)
0 to 1	1.8	4.0	-2.2*
2	12.3	7.4	4.9
≥3	24.2	9.9	14.3

*Negative sign indicates increase in risk.

      b.   Male sex

      c.   History of hemispheric transient ischemic attack or stroke

      d.   Intermittent claudication

      e.   80% to 94% internal carotid artery stenosis

      f.   No collateral circulation (cerebral angiography)

   v.   Table 16-5 summarizes impact of these risk factors in patients experiencing TMVL

E.   Ischemic ocular syndrome

   1.   Chronic hypoperfusion of the globe from ipsilateral or bilateral carotid occlusive disease

   2.   Subdivide findings (Table 16-6)

      a.   Anterior segment ischemia

      b.   Hypoperfusion retinopathy

   3.   Ischemic uveitis is nonresponsive to topical corticosteroid drops

Table 16-6

FINDINGS IN OCULAR ISCHEMIC SYNDROME

Conjunctiva
Injected vessels
Dilated episcleral vessels

Cornea
Edema

Anterior chamber
Cells, flare (ischemic uveitis)

Iris
Neovascularization
± Increased intraocular pressure

Pupil
Sluggish
Afferent defect

Lens
Cataract

Retina
Dilated arterioles
Dilated venules
Microaneurysms
Retinal hemorrhages
Neovascularization
Vitreous hemorrhage
Traction retinal detachment
Fluorescein angiography: decreased filling
and increased transit time

4.   Hypoperfusion retinopathy, also known as venous stasis retinopathy, occurs three to four times more commonly than anterior segment ischemia
5.   Retinopathy: dot-and-blot hemorrhages typically located in midperiphery
6.   Treatment
    a.   Ocular neovascularization: intravitreal anti-VEGF (vascular endothelial growth factor) agent; panretinal photocoagulation
    b.   Medical and surgical therapy to improve carotid artery flow to the eye
7.   5-year mortality: 40%

F.   Internal carotid artery dissection
    1.   Leads to ischemia due to decreased blood flow or distal embolization
    2.   Cause of stroke in young patients (<50 years)
    3.   Etiology:
        a.   Spontaneous
        b.   Traumatic
        c.   Arterial wall disease (pseudoxanthoma elasticum, fibrous dysplasia, Ehlers-Danlos syndrome)
    4.   Ocular involvement:
        a.   Horner's syndrome (see Chapter 8)
        b.   TMVL
        c.   Ischemic optic neuropathy
        d.   CRAO
        e.   Ocular motor cranial nerve palsy

   5.   Associated symptoms:
        a.   Headache
        b.   Neck pain
        c.   Tinnitus
        d.   Dysgeusia
G.   Ocular motor cranial nerve palsies
     1.   Very rare association with carotid thrombosis or dissection
     2.   Ocular pain
     3.   Ipsilateral blindness
     4.   III, IV, VI nerve palsies last 6 to 24 hours
     5.   Thrombosis of branches of ophthalmic artery supplying orbital branches of III, IV, VI nerves causes ophthalmoplegia; transient because collateral flow is able to restore perfusion to ocular motor nerves (see Figure 16-1)

BIBLIOGRAPHY

Books

Bernstein EF, ed. *Amaurosis Fugax*. New York, NY: Springer-Verlag; 1988.

Chapters

Biousse, V. Cerebrovascular diseases. In: Miller NR, Newman NJ, eds. *Walsh and Hoyt's Clinical Neuro-Ophthalmology*. 6th ed. Vol 7. Baltimore, Md: Williams & Wilkins; 2005:1967-2168.

Burde RM, Savino PJ, Trobe JD. *Clinical Decisions in Neuro-Ophthalmology*. 3rd ed. St Louis, Mo: Mosby-Year Book; 2002:94-113.

Digre KB, Corbett JJ. *Practical Viewing of the Optic Disc*. Boston, Mass: Butterworth-Heinemann; 2003:269-344.

Articles

Benavente O, Eliasiw W, Streifler JY, et al. Prognosis after transient monocular blindness associated with carotid-artery stenosis. *N Engl J Med*. 2001;345:1084-1090.

Biousse V. The coagulation system. *J Neuroophthalmol*. 2003;23:50-62.

Biousse V, Trobe JD. Treatment monocular visual loss. *Am J Ophthalmol*. 2003;140:717-722.

Carter JE. Carotid artery disease and its ocular manifestations. *Ophthalmol Clin North Am*. 1992;5:425-443.

European Carotid Surgery Trialists Collaborative Group. Risk of stroke in the distribution of an asymptomatic carotid artery. *Lancet*. 1995;345:209-212.

Executive Committee for the Asymptomatic Carotid Atherosclerosis Study. Endarterectomy for asymptomatic carotid stenosis. *JAMA*. 1995;275:1421-1428.

Fisher CM. Observation of the fundus oculi in transient monocular blindness. *Neurology*. 1959;9:333-347.

Hayreh SS, Kolder HE, Weingeist TA. Central retinal artery occlusion and retinal tolerance time. *Ophthalmology*. 1980;87:75-78.

Hollenhorst RS. Significance of bright plaques in the retinal arterioles. *JAMA*. 1961;178:23-29.

Kearns TP, Hollenhorst R. Venous-stasis retinopathy of occlusive disease of the carotid artery. *Proceedings of the Staff Meetings of the Mayo Clinic*. 1963;38:304-312.

Lorentzen SE. Occlusion of the central retinal artery: a follow-up. *Acta Ophthalmol.* 1969;47:690-703.

North American Symptomatic Carotid Endarterectomy Trial Collaborators. Beneficial effect of carotid endarterectomy in symptomatic patients with high-grade carotid stenosis. *N Engl J Med.* 1991;325:445-453.

Trobe JD. Who needs carotid endarterectomy (circa 1996)? *Ophthalmol Clin North Am.* 1996;9:513-519.

Chapter 17

Non-Organic Visual Disorders

Richard H. Fish, MD, FACS

I. **Definitions and historical perspective**

    A.   Non-organic visual disorders

        1.   No physiologic or organic basis

        2.   Also termed: functional, nonphysiologic

        3.   Classically divided into two main groups:

            a.   Hysteria

            b.   Malingering

        4.   These two groups cannot always be differentiated; rather form a spectrum of disease

    B.   Malingering: willfully misleading the existence or seriousness of a disease or disability for the purpose of a consciously desired end

        1.   Duke-Elder: "Common manifestation of human weakness ... wicked or lazy"

        2.   Keltner: California syndrome—economic gain from visual loss. Estimated $300 million paid in 1982 for fraudulent workers' compensation claims

    C.   Hysteria (Greek: "condition of the womb"): also known as conversion disorder. Subconscious expression of symptoms without demonstrable organic findings, usually involving loss or alteration of sensorimotor functions. Symptoms may have underlying symbolic meaning and are often precipitated by psychological stress or physical trauma

        1.   Referred to in Egyptian papyri, writings of Hippocrates, and in the New Testament of the Bible

        2.   Plato: unfulfilled uterus wandering about the body

        3.   Charcot: "dissociation of vision" caused by lesion in brain

        4.   Babinski: "pithiatism"; disorders caused by suggestion and cured by persuasion

        5.   Freud: sexual pleasure in looking (scopophilia); results in repression of forbidden sights into the unconscious with the eyes now "at the disposal of the repressed sexual instinct and hence unable to function properly"

    D.   Differentiating malingering from hysteria

1. Malingerer will exaggerate symptoms ("blinder than the blind"), while hysterics are classically described as having "la belle indifference" to their affliction

2. Hysterical patients tend to be cooperative; malingerers irritable and combative, especially with prolonged testing

3. Malingering usually involves secondary gain (eg, financial reward or avoiding military service). Hysterics may receive secondary gain in the form of attention

II. Evaluation: in assessing patients with non-organic visual disorders, learn a few tests well and be able to perform them quickly and naturally

A. Total binocular blindness

1. Observation: truly blind moves cautiously, bumps into things naturally; hysteric avoids objects, "seeing unconsciously"; malingerer goes out of his or her way to bump into objects

2. Pupillary response: easiest and single most important test

a. Intact direct and consensual responses exclude anterior visual pathway disease (don't forget about pharmacologic mydriasis in a malingerer)

b. In patients with vision better than no light perception (NLP), there is no consistent relationship between amount of visual loss and pupillary deficit

3. Menace reflex: blinking to visual threat

4. Sudden strong illumination. Difficult to suppress reflex tearing

5. Signature: truly blind have no difficulty. Functionally blind sign their name with exaggerated illegibility

6. Looking at hand or touching index fingers together depends on proprioception, not vision. Blind have no trouble with this; malingerers, thinking that these tasks require good vision, will perform poorly

7. Optokinetic nystagmus (OKN): difficult but possible to suppress. Optimum response obtained when rate of succession of object is 3 to 12 per second

8. Mirror tracking: eyes move in response to the image in a mirror as it is rocked back and forth. Mirror must be large enough to prevent patient from looking around it (approximately 33 x 67 cm)

9. Making sudden ridiculous facial expressions. Results in "considerable loss of dignity...and residents falling into an acute fit of choking" (Thompson, 1985)

10. Visual evoked response: flash and pattern-reversal stimuli. Correlation exists between check size and level of acuity. Although difficult, it is possible to consciously alter response to pattern-reversal stimulation with convergence, meditation, and intense concentration

B. Total monocular blindness: more common than binocular. Can use any of the above tests with unaffected eyes occluded

1. Diplopia tests

a. Suspected eye is occluded while a strong prism is held with the apex bisecting the pupil of the good eye. Patient admits to monocular diplopia. As the suspected eye is uncovered, the entire prism is placed before the good eye, producing binocular diplopia. If the patient still reports diplopia, functional blindness is revealed

   b. Have the patient walk up and down stairs with a vertical prism over the allegedly blind eye

  2. Fixation tests

   a. Ten-diopter base-out test: relies upon refixation movements to avoid diplopia. Ten-diopter base-out prism in front of a normal eye produces shift of both eyes with a refixation movement of the other eye. A truly blind eye will not refixate, and a prism placed before this eye should result in no movement of either eye

   b. Vertical bar: ruler held 5 inches from the nose in between the eyes while the patient reads at near. Overlap of visual fields allows a binocular person to read across the bar without interruption. A truly monocular patient will pause to shift fixation across the bar. If the patient reads without interruption, functional blindness is confirmed. Can also use a prism in front of the suspected eye, resulting in diplopia that should interrupt reading

  3. Fogging tests

   a. Both eyes are open in a phoropter; the patient begins reading the eye chart. Examiner progressively adds more plus to the good eye while the patient keeps reading. Final line read is the patient's acuity in the suspected eye

   b. Crossed cylinder technique: two strong cylindrical lenses of equal power—plus and minus—are placed at the same axis in the trial frame over the sound eye. Patient reads with both eyes open and the examiner, pretending to make an adjustment, rotates one lens 45 degrees, fogging the good eye

   c. Instill a cycloplegic agent into the unaffected eye; have the patient read at near

  4. Color tests

   a. Red/green duochrome in the projector, red/green glasses worn such that the red lens covers the suspected eye. Eye behind the red lens sees letters on red and not green side of the chart; eye behind the green lens sees only letters on the green side. If the patient reads the entire line, the suspected eye is being used

   b. Red/green glasses and Worth four-dot test. Patient should see appropriate number of dots

   c. Polaroid glasses and vectographic slides: each eye sees different portions of the eye chart. If the patient reads entire line, both eyes are being utilized

  5. Stereoscopic tests: stereoacuity is directly proportional to Snellen acuity—40 seconds of arc stereoacuity compatible with no worse than 20/20 Snellen acuity OU

C. Diminished vision: simulation of visual acuity less than 20/20. More difficult to detect. May be binocular or monocular. Can use most of the tests above, plus the following:

  1. DKR ("doctor killing refraction") or toothpaste refraction ("squeeze it out of them"): start with 20/10 line and express disbelief that the patient could not see the huge letters on the 20/15 line, then proceed up the chart until the patient reads

2. Visual angle: varying test distances with eye chart, Landolt C rings or Tumbling E block such that the patient sees a smaller visual angle or demonstrates inconsistencies (eg, reading 20/20 letters at 10 feet is equivalent to 20/40 acuity)

3. Move the patient back and forth slightly in the chair, helping him or her "get into focus" or place combinations of lenses adding up to plano in a trial frame to help magnify the vision

III. Conditions misdiagnosed as non-organic visual loss

A. Keratoconus: biomicroscopy, K readings, corneal topography

B. Amblyopia: look for strabismus, anisometropia

C. Early Stargardt's disease: macular examination, fluorescein angiography

D. Retinitis pigmentosa sine pigmento: electroretinography (ERG)

E. Central serous chorioretinopathy: macular examination, fluorescein angiography

F. Cystoid macular edema: ophthalmoscopy, fluorescein angiography, optical coherence tomography (OCT)

G. Cone dystrophy: ERG

H. Paraneoplastic retinopathy: ERG, systemic evaluation

I. Bilateral occipital lobe infarctions: magnetic resonance imaging (MRI)

IV. Other non-organic eye diseases

A. Visual field loss

1. Monocular visual field defects

   a. Concentric contraction with no expansion of the field at an increasing test distance (tunnel vision, see Figure 1-24 and Chapter 1 for differential diagnosis of markedly constricted visual fields)

   b. Spiraling isopters (Figure 17-1)

   c. Crossing isopters (Figure 17-2)

   d. These same visual field defects have also been reported in patients with frontal lobe tumors

   e. Monocular temporal hemianopia that persists on binocular testing (Figure 17-3)

2. Binocular visual field defects

   a. Normal binocular perimetry: visual field performed with both eyes open measures approximately 180 degrees in width with no blind spots due to overlap of monocular fields

   b. Monocular visual field subtends approximately 150 degrees, with a greater field temporally due to unpaired temporal crescent (see Chapter 1)

   c. True monocular blindness: binocular perimetry demonstrates blind spot of a normal eye with loss of the temporal crescent of the blind eye (Figure 17-4)

   d. Non-organic monocular blindness: binocular perimetry reveals a full visual field (Figure 17-5)

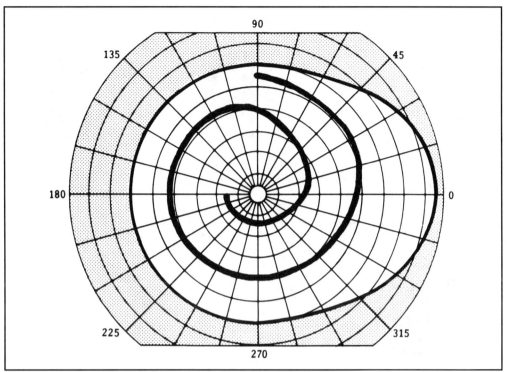

Figure 17-1. Spiraling isopters.

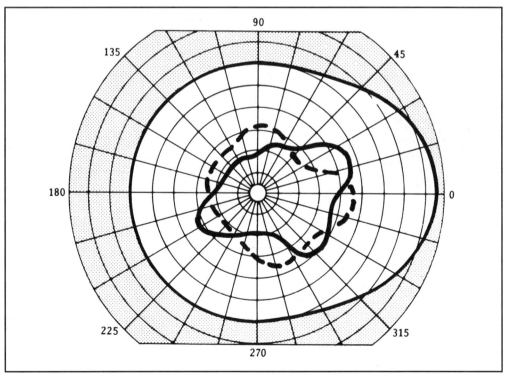

Figure 17-2. Crossing isopters.

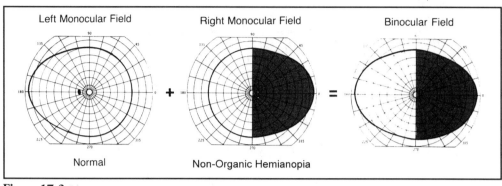

Figure 17-3.

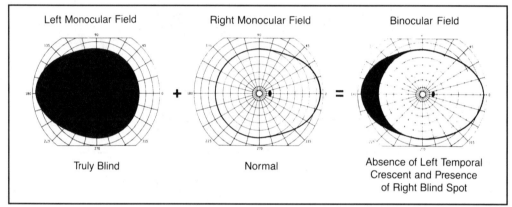

Figure 17-4.

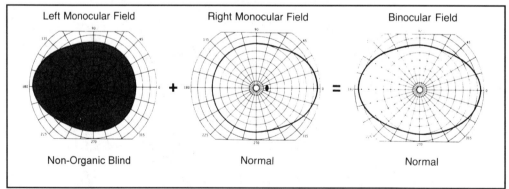

Figure 17-5.

e. Non-organic bitemporal hemianopia: patients with true bitemporal hemianopia have a binocular field composed of two nasal hemifields (Figure 17-6). With non-organic bitemporal hemianopia, the patient claims inability to see temporally, with only a thin island of vision straddling the vertical midline (Figure 17-7)

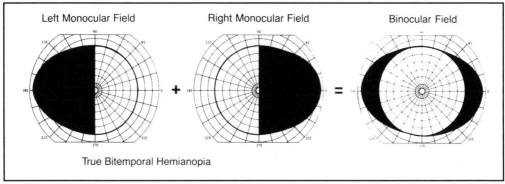

Figure 17-6.

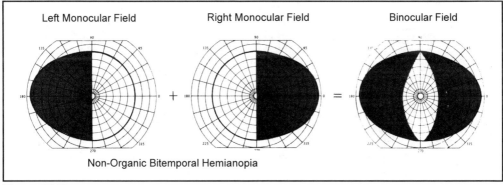

Figure 17-7.

f.   Binasal hemianopia: rare. Usually due to optic nerve or retinal disease (glaucoma, disc drusen, chronic papilledema, retinoschisis, retinal detachment, chorioretinal degeneration). Intracranial causes include basilar skull fracture, neurosyphilis, chiasmal arachnoiditis, and neoplasm. Binasal defects of organic etiology are seldom complete and rarely respect the vertical midline. If defects are complete, there is "prefixation blindness" (Figure 17-8)

g.   Caution: automated perimetry cannot differentiate non-organic from organic visual field loss. Malingerers can simulate neurologic field defects when tested with an automated visual field machine

B.   Voluntary nystagmus
1.   Irregular brief bursts of rapid frequency, low amplitude, horizontal pendular eye movements; actually back-to-back saccades
2.   Up to 8% of normal individuals can produce this
3.   Usually bilateral and conjugate
4.   May be associated with convergence, fluttering eyelids, blinking, or strained facial expression
5.   Oscillopsia common

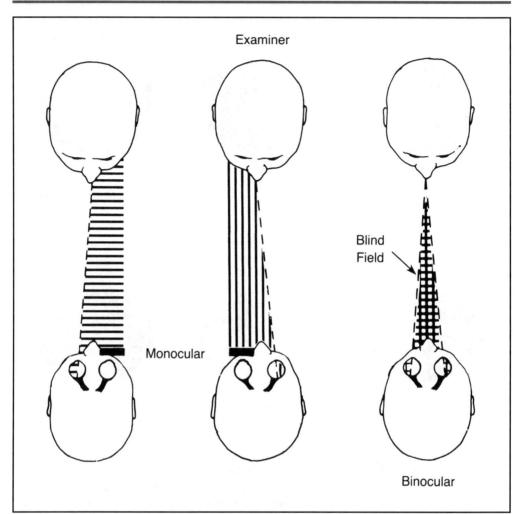

Figure 17-8. Binasal hemianopia. Monocular testing reveals hemianopic field defects nasal to the visual axis in each eye. With organic etiology, binocular testing confirms blindness in the area where the two nasal hemifields overlap (prefixation blindness). An object moving through this area will suddenly disappear and reappear. (Modified from Thompson HS. Binasal field loss. In: Thompson HS, ed. *Topics in Neuro-Ophthalmology.* Baltimore, Md: Williams & Wilkins; 1979:84.)

6.   The initiation of nystagmus is under voluntary control, while rate, amplitude, and duration of nystagmus are not
7.   Difficult to maintain longer than 10 to 20 seconds
8.   May be familial

C.   Accommodative spasm
   1.   Relatively common
   2.   Intermittent episodes of convergence associated with miosis, accommodation, and induced myopia
   3.   Pupils constrict on attempted lateral gaze (Figure 17-9)
   4.   No abduction deficit with oculocephalic (doll's eye) or caloric testing

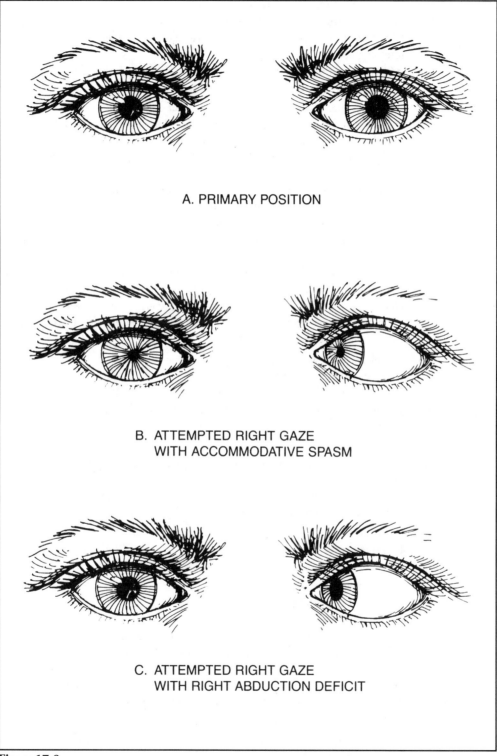

A. PRIMARY POSITION

B. ATTEMPTED RIGHT GAZE
WITH ACCOMMODATIVE SPASM

C. ATTEMPTED RIGHT GAZE
WITH RIGHT ABDUCTION DEFICIT

Figure 17-9.

      5.   May have diplopia and micropsia

      6.   May be interrupted by patching or cycloplegia

      7.   Differential diagnosis includes VI nerve palsy and other conditions causing limited abduction (see Chapter 4)

      8.   Treatment is difficult; may involve atropine drops and bifocals; medial rectus injection with botulinum toxin

D.   Monocular diplopia: usually non-organic cause but occasionally organic

      1.   External causes: chalazion; eyelid tumor at ridge of corneal epithelium; mucus strand, vegetable fiber, or oil droplet in tear film

      2.   Optical causes: irregular astigmatism; keratoconus; tilted or subluxed lens; lens clefts, vacuoles, or cataracts; gas bubbles, glass, crystals, parasite larvae in vitreous; macular cysts; epimacular membrane, central serous chorioretinopathy, diabetic macular edema causes distortion, not diplopia

      3.   Neurologic causes: rare. Reported in pituitary tumor, tumor or hemorrhage of occipital cortex, lesions in frontal eye field controlling voluntary eye movement

      4.   Transiently seen following strabismus surgery in patients with anomalous retinal correspondence

      5.   Diagnosis: pinhole usually eliminates optical causes. Careful retinoscopy and biomicroscopy is essential. Contact lenses may be useful in correcting about 60% of cases of monocular diplopia

E.   Voluntary blepharospasm

      1.   May be unilateral or bilateral

      2.   May resemble ptosis or true blepharospasm

      3.   Isolated or associated with functional decreased vision or accommodative spasm

F.   Non-organic asthenopia

      1.   Complaints of painful sensations in and around the eyes, lacrimation, photophobia

      2.   Inability to read without headache or eyestrain despite correction of refractive error and normal muscle balance

G.   Voluntary gaze palsy

      1.   Infrequently seen

      2.   Limitation of upgaze

          a.   Lack of cooperation

          b.   Normal aging phenomenon

          c.   Non-organic etiology

          d.   Rule out dorsal midbrain syndrome (see Chapter 2)

      3.   Paralysis of horizontal gaze: one case report of a patient unable to make saccadic or pursuit movements to the left. Examiners were unable to overcome "paralysis" with oculocephalic (doll's eye) testing, OKN, or mirror tracking. Also noted were convergence and miosis on attempted left gaze

H.   Ocular Münchausen's syndrome

      1.   Deliberate deception by a patient involving fabricated medical histories, self-inflicted physical abnormalities, and self-mutilation

2. Reported ocular manifestations include voluntary nystagmus; subconjunctival hemorrhage; conjunctivitis; pharmacologic mydriasis; corneal erosion, ulcer, and alkali burn; self-induced chronic orbital cellulitis requiring exenteration; and chronic periorbital abscess

3. Psychiatric evaluation mandatory, but treatment is frequently unsuccessful

I. Non-organic chromatopsia or micropsia

V. Natural history of non-organic visual loss

A. Twenty-seven percent of patients demonstrated a chronic course with no improvement of visual acuity (Friesen & Mann, 1966)

B. Twelve percent of patients eventually found to have macular disease (Rada et al, 1973)

C. Twenty-three of 42 patients (55%) continued to have functional visual loss when followed 16 to 156 months (mean: 53 months). Few were socially or economically impaired despite persistent visual loss (Kathol et al, 1983)

D. Seventy-two percent of 46 patients younger than 21 years of age showed improvement in non-organic visual field loss (Murata & Takahashi, 1993)

E. Beware of the patient with both organic and non-organic disease. A follow-up study of 85 patients with a variety of conversion disorders (Slater & Glithero, 1965) found that:

1. Twenty-two patients were found to have coexistent organic diseases, including generalized disease of the central nervous system

2. Two patients subsequently developed schizophrenia

3. Four patients committed suicide

4. Eight patients died of organic disease that was present at the time of diagnosis of "hysteria"

VI. Treatment of non-organic eye disease

A. Reassurance that the problem will get better, emphasizing positive things that the eye does well—peripheral vision, normal pupils, optic nerve, retina, etc

B. Do not use eye drops, orthoptic exercises, or spectacles. This draws attention to the eyes and undermines reassurance

C. Confrontation is rarely productive

D. Psychiatric consultation

E. "Retinal rest": hospitalized with bilateral patches and sensory deprivation (no radio, TV, visitors, etc)

BIBLIOGRAPHY

Chapters

Freud S. The psycho-analytic view of psychogenic disturbances of vision. In: *The Standard Edition of the Complete Psychological Works of Sigmund Freud*. London: Hogarth Press; 1957:XI,211-218.

Kline LB. Techniques for diagnosis functional visual loss. In: Parrish RK, ed. *The University of Miami Bascom Palmer Eye Institute Atlas of Ophthalmology*. Boston, Mass: Butterworth-Heinemann; 2000:493-501.

Miller NR. Neuro-ophthalmologic manifestations of nonorganic disease. In: Miller NR, Newman NJ, eds. *Walsh and Hoyt's Clinical Neuro-Ophthalmology*. 6th ed. Vol 1. Philadelphia, Pa: Lippincott Williams & Wilkins; 2005:1315-1334.

Articles

Bumgartner J, Epstein CM. Voluntary alteration of visual evoked potentials. *Ann Neurol*. 1982;12:475-478.

Caplan LR, Nadelson T. Multiple sclerosis and hysteria. Lessons learned from their association. *JAMA*. 1980;24:2418-2421.

Friesen H, Mann WA. Follow-up study of hysterical amblyopia. *Am J Ophthalmol*. 1966;62:1106-1115.

Goldstein JH, Schneekloth B. Spasm of the near reflex: a spectrum of anomalies. *Surv Ophthalmol*. 1996;40:269-278.

Kathol RG, Cox TA, Corbett JJ, et al. Functional visual loss. II. Psychiatric aspects in 42 patients followed for 4 years. *Psychol Med*. 1983;13:315-324.

Keane JR. Hysterical hemianopia. The "missing half" defect. *Arch Ophthalmol*. 1979;97:865-866.

Keltner JL, May WN, Johnson CA, et al. The California syndrome. Functional visual complaints with potential economic impact. *Ophthalmology*. 1985;92:427-435.

Kramer KK, La Piana FG, Appleton B. Ocular malingering and hysteria: diagnosis and management. *Surv Ophthalmol*. 1979;24:89-96.

Lim SA, Siatkowski RM, Farris BK. Functional visual loss in adults and children. *Ophthalmology*. 2005;112:1821-1828.

McIntyre A. Spasm of the near reflex: a literature review. *British Orthoptic Journal*. 2001;58:3-11.

Murata M, Takahashi S. Psychogenic visual disturbances in patients under 21 years of age. *Folia Ophthalmology of Japan*. 1993;44:53-58.

Rada RT, Krill AE, Meyer GG, et al. Visual conversion reaction in children II. Followup. *Psychosomatics*. 1973;14:271-276.

Rosenberg PN, Krohel GB, Webb RM, et al. Ocular Münchausen's syndrome. *Ophthalmology*. 1986;93:1120-1123.

Scott JA, Egan RA. Prevalence of organic neuro-ophthalmologic disease in patients with functional visual loss. *Am J Ophthalmol*. 2003;135:670-675.

Slater E, Glithero E. A follow-up of patients diagnosed as suffering from hysteria. *J Psychosom Res*. 1965;9:9-13.

Stewart JFG. Automated perimetry and malingerers. *Ophthalmology*. 1995;102:27-32.

Troost BT, Troost EG. Functional paralysis of horizontal gaze. *Neurology*. 1979;29:82-85.

Chapter 18

Disorders of Higher Visual Function

Christopher A. Girkin, MD, MSPH, FACS

I. **Anatomical considerations**

   A. Information concerning different aspects of visual perception is conveyed to the striate cortex through at least three distinct pathways: parvocellular, magnocellular, and koniocellular (see below)

   B. From the striate cortex, this information is further analyzed by several functionally distinct visual associative areas in and adjacent to the occipital lobes to further refine the incoming information (Figures 18-1 and 18-2)

   C. From these associative areas, two occipitofugal pathways project to other cortical areas involved in higher order processing of visual perceptual information (Figure 18-3)

   D. Damage to these areas may cause selective loss of isolated components of visual perception yielding an array of perceptual abnormalities that have localizing value to the clinician

II. **Overview of the visual system**

   A. Retinogeniculate pathways:

   1. Over 22 types of ganglion cells exist in the primate retina. While other ganglion cells project to numerous subcortical nuclei, primarily three types of ganglion cells appear to be involved in visual perception and project to specific locations within the lateral geniculate nucleus (LGN)

   2. Parvocellular pathway

      a. Originates in the midget ganglion cell in the retina; these cells have small receptive fields tuned to fine spatial resolution

      b. Conveys information concerning red-green opponency

      c. Static firing system—not keyed to detect motion

      d. Ring or High Pass Resolution perimetry and spatial contrast sensitivity test this pathway

   3. Magnocellular pathway

      a. Originates in the parasol ganglion cells in the retina, which have large receptive fields and low spatial resolution

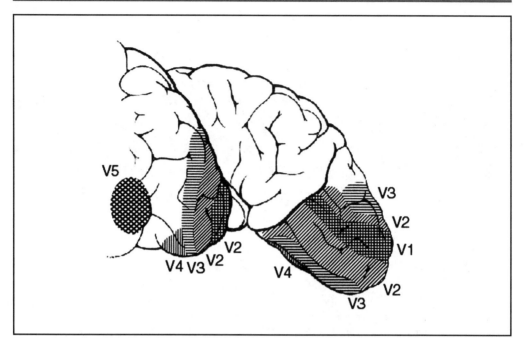

Figure 18-1. Posterior lateral view of the human visual cortex showing the clinically relevant visual associative areas. The cerebellum has been removed and the hemispheres have been separated and displaced to display medial and lateral occipital regions. V1 corresponds to the primary or striate visual cortex.

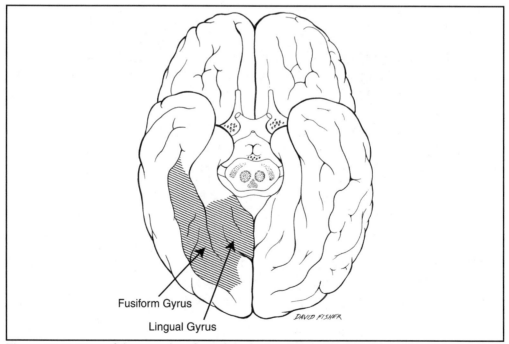

Figure 18-2. View of the ventral surface of the brain with the cerebellum removed. The posterior fusiform and lingual gyri contain the human color center.

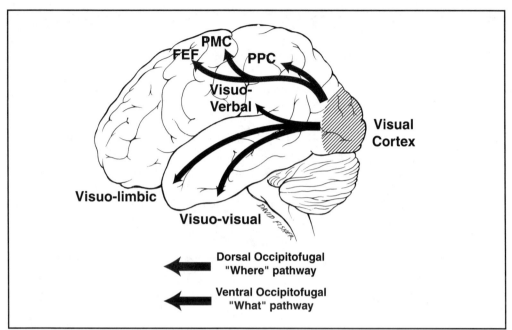

Figure 18-3. Parallel visual processing pathways in the human. The ventral, or "what," pathway begins in the striate cortex (V1) and projects to the angular gyrus for language processing, the inferior temporal lobe for object identification and limbic structures. The dorsal, or "where," pathway begins in the striate cortex and projects to the posterior parietal and superior temporal cortex, dealing with visuospatial analysis. (FEF=frontal eye field, PMC=premotor cortex, PPC=posterior parietal cortex.)

        b.   Conveys information concerning motion

        c.   Phasic firing system—keyed to motion detection

        d.   Frequency doubled perimetry and motion-automated perimetry were designed to emphasize the response characteristics of this pathway

    4.   Koniocellular pathway

        a.   Originates from the bistratified ganglion cells in the retina, which have large receptive fields and low spatial resolution

        b.   Conveys information concerning blue-yellow spectral opponency

        c.   Short wavelength automated perimetry (SWAP) was designed to emphasize the response characteristics of this pathway

B.   Specialized visual cortical areas

    1.   Over the past 20 years, more than 30 visual cortical areas have been isolated in macaque monkeys. These areas comprise almost 50% of the entire cortical volume

    2.   The visual cortex in the macaque was initially divided into six subregions, named visual areas 1 through 6 (areas V1 to V6) which incompletely surround the striate cortex (see Figure 18-1)

    3.   Area V1 is the primary visual cortex and corresponds to the striate cortex in both humans and lower primates (area 17)

    4.   Areas V2 to V6 form concentric bands that incompletely surround area V1

Table 18-1

LESION OF ASSOCIATIVE VISUAL AREAS

1. Area V1
   a. Anton's syndrome
   b. Blindsight
   c. Riddoch's phenomenon
   d. Visual ataxia
2. Areas V2 and V3
   a. Quadrantic homonymous hemianopia
3. Area V4
   a. Cerebral achromatopsia
4. Area V5
   a. Akinetopsia

5. Five important cortical visual areas in man (see Figures 18-1 and 18-2)
   a. V1 or striate cortex
   b. V2 and V3—surrounds the striate cortex
   c. V4—in the ventromedial occipital lobe involved in color perception
   d. V5—in the lateral occipital lobe involved in motion perception
6. Damage to these areas may yield a variety of visual disturbances (Table 18-1)

C. Two occipitofugal pathways convey information from the occipital lobe to more anterior visual associative areas (see Figure 18-3)
   1. Dorsal occipitofugal pathway or "where" pathway
      a. Projections involved in visuospatial analysis, in the localization of objects in visual space, and in modulation of visual guidance of movements toward these objects
      b. Begins in V1 and projects through V2 and V3 to V5. From V5, this pathway continues to the parietal and superior temporal cortex
      c. Lesions of this pathway cause visuospatial disorders, such as simultanagnosia, optic ataxia, acquired oculomotor apraxia, and hemispatial neglect
   2. Ventral occipitofugal pathway or "what" pathway
      a. Projections involved in processing the physical attributes of a visual image that are important to the perception of color, shape, and pattern
      b. Information is crucial for object identification and object-based attention and provides visual information to areas involved in visual identification, language processing, memory, and emotion
      c. Originates in V1 and projects through V2 and V4 to specific inferior temporal cortical areas, the angular gyrus, and limbic structures
      d. Lesions in this pathway may cause a variety of associative defects including visual alexia and anomia, visual agnosia, visual amnesia, and visual hypoemotionality

III.   Syndromes associated with damage to the striate cortex (area V1)

    A.   Anton's syndrome

        1.   Definition: denial of blindness, which usually occurs following bilateral damage to the striate cortex

        2.   Occasionally seen with prechiasmal blindness

        3.   Possible causes:

            a.   Damage to higher cognitive centers

            b.   Psychiatric denial

            c.   Disruption of pathways from visual areas to cerebral regions involved with conscious awareness

    B.   Blindsight

        1.   Definition: unconscious rudimentary visual perception that may persist in blind patients following lesions to the visual cortex

        2.   Multiple levels of preserved function

            a.   Subcortical (reflexive) blindsight:

                i.   Preserved visual-neuroendocrine response due to retino-hypothalamic connections

                ii.   Preservation of the photic blink reflex

                iii.   Preservation of OKNs reported in one patient with cortical blindness

            b.   Higher level preserved visual responses in a blind hemifield

                i.   Unconscious detection of stimulus presence, type, orientation, motion, and wavelength has been described

        3.   Possibly due to pathways through the superior colliculus that bypass the damaged striate cortex, or due to connections between the LGN to extrastriatal visual cortical areas

        4.   While these residual abilities may be enhanced with practice, the role of blindsight in visual rehabilitation is controversial

    C.   Riddoch phenomenon (statokinetic dissociation)

        1.   Definition: preservation of perception of motion in an otherwise blind hemifield

        2.   Possible causes:

            a.   Activation of extrastriate areas (V5)

            b.   Residual island of function in the striate cortex

            c.   Lateral summation of moving images (may be seen in normals)

        3.   Clinically, the presence of Riddoch's phenomena in a hemianopic defect following an occipital stroke is a good prognostic sign that the visual field will improve

    D.   Visual ataxia

        1.   Definition: patients with homonymous hemianopia from occipital lobe lesions may experience loss of balance with the sensation of falling toward their blind hemifield

        2.   Patients have normal vestibular responses, and the "visual ataxia" is thought to be due to unopposed input from the contralateral intact visual cortex

Table 18-2

CAUSES OF CENTRAL ACHROMATOPSIA

1. Bilateral posterior cerebral artery infarction
2. Metastatic tumor involving the ventromedial occipital cortex
3. Posterior cortical dementia
4. Herpes simplex encephalitis involving the ventromedial occipital cortex
5. Seizure disorder (transient)
6. Migraine (transient)
7. Vertebrobasilar insufficiency (transient)

IV. Syndromes caused by damage to the parastriate and peristriate visual cortex (V2 and V3)

    A.   Quadrantic homonymous hemianopia that respects the horizontal meridian may occur with lesions of V2 and V3 based on magnetic resonance imaging (MRI) correlations presumably due to the greater separation of the superior and inferior fields in these regions

V. Syndromes caused by damage to the human color center

    A.   Cerebral achromatopsia

        1.   Definition: loss of color perception due to damage to the ventromedial occipital cortex, posterior lingual, and fusiform gyri (see Figure 18-2)

        2.   Etiology (Table 18-2)

        3.   Bilateral lesions may cause complete achromatopsia; unilateral lesions will cause hemiachromatopsia

        4.   Often associated with superior visual field defects and disorders of the ventral occipitofugal pathway (see below)

VI. Syndromes caused by damage to area V5

    A.   Akinetopsia

        1.   Definition: loss of perception of visual motion with preservation of the perception of other modalities of vision, such as form, texture, and color

        2.   Caused by bilateral lesions of the ventrolateral occipital gyri (see area V5 in Figure 18-1)

            a.   Only two cases due to cerebral infarctions following sagittal sinus thrombosis have been extensively studied

            b.   Subtle deficits in motion processing have been demonstrated in the contralateral hemifield in patients with unilateral damage to this area

VII. Syndromes of the dorsal occipitofugal pathway in humans

    A.   Simultanagnosia

        1.   Definition: failure to integrate multiple elements of a visual scene into one global image

        2.   Patients with simultanagnosia can only attend to one element of a visual scene at a time and describe only fragments of a picture, despite intact visual fields

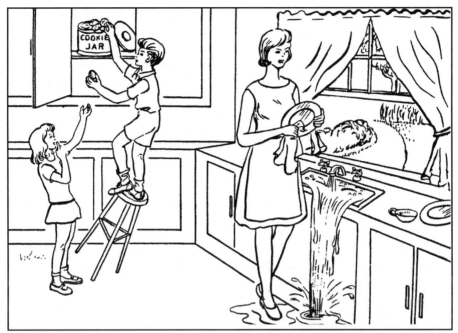

Figure 18-4. The "cookie theft picture," modified from the Boston Diagnostic Aphasia Examination. This picture contains a balance of information among the four visual field quadrants. A patient is asked to describe the events in the picture, a task that requires assimilation of the entire visual scene.

      3.   The cookie theft picture is an excellent test for simultanagnosia (Figure 18-4)

      4.   Due to lesions of the posterior parietal cortex (PPC)

           a.   Stroke (especially watershed infraction)

           b.   Tumors

           c.   Encephalitis

           d.   Alzheimer's disease

           e.   Posterior cortical dementia

B.   Optic ataxia

      1.   Definition: a disorder of visual guidance of movements in which visual inputs are disconnected from the motor systems; thus, patients with an intact field reach for targets as if they were blind

      2.   Etiology: a complex sensory-motor network involving the PPC, premotor cortex, motor areas, ventromedial cortical areas, and subcortical structures, such as the cerebellum, that modulate the control of visually guided limb movement. Any lesion that disrupts this network can cause optic ataxia

      3.   As a rule, lesions of the superior parietal cortex are more likely to damage areas involved with limb guidance, whereas inferior parietal lesions are more likely to affect visual attention and thus produce neglect syndromes

C.   Acquired ocular motor apraxia (spasm of fixation)

      1.   Definition: loss of voluntary eye movements with persistence of fixation on a target. In contrast to true ocular motor apraxia seen in childhood, saccades are easily made to peripheral targets in the absence of a fixation target

2.   Etiology: damage to the frontal eye field (FEF) inhibits the release of fixation

D.   Hemispatial (hemifield) neglect
1.   Definition: a visuospatial disorder in which patients are unable to attend to stimuli presented into the left hemifield, despite full visual fields
2.   Caused by damage to a network in the right hemisphere that controls visuospatial attention to both hemispheres. These areas include:
   a.   PPC—builds the sensory representation of extrapersonal space
   b.   FEF—plans and initiates exploratory movements
   c.   Cingulate gyrus—provides motivational potential
3.   Hemispatial neglect may appear as a left homonymous hemianopia on double simultaneous confrontational field testing. Presenting stimuli to one side at a time will reveal intact areas in the left visual field that are masked with bilateral testing
4.   Since the right cerebral hemisphere may mediate attention in both hemifields, right-sided hemineglect does not occur with left hemispheric lesions

E.   Visual allesthesia
1.   Definition: a disorder of visuospatial perception in which the retinotopic visual field is rotated, flipped, or even inverted
2.   Causative lesion may disturb the integration of visual and otolithic inputs at the level of the medulla or at the site of integration in the PPC
3.   Etiology (Table 18-3)

VIII. Lesions of the ventral occipitofugal pathway in humans

A.   Visual-verbal disconnection
1.   Definition: these syndromes are due to disconnection of visual input to areas in the dominant angular gyrus, which deals with language processing; thus, patients have difficulty naming objects from sight
2.   Etiology: most commonly seen with left occipital infarctions that also damages fibers crossing in the splenium of the corpus collosum carrying visual information from the right hemisphere to left-sided language areas
3.   Types:
   a.   Alexia without agraphia—loss of the ability to read with preservation of writing ability
   b.   Color anomia—loss of the ability to name colors with preservation of color matching (ie, color perception is normal)
   c.   Optic anomia—generalized deficit in the ability to name visual objects or categories of objects

B.   Visual-visual disconnection
1.   Definition: these syndromes develop due to disconnection of visual information from occipital areas to areas within the temporal lobe involved in object identification
2.   Etiology: usually results from bilateral damage to the inferior portions of the occipitotemporal cortex, notably the lingual and fusiform gyri
3.   Types:
   a.   Prosopagnosia—loss of the ability to visually identify previously familiar faces. Identification by other sensory (eg, voice, mannerisms) modalities remain intact

Table 18-3

Etiology of Visual Hallucinations and Illusions

I.   Visual hallucinations
    A.   Psychiatric disorders
        1.   Schizophrenia
        2.   Narcolepsy
        3.   Psychotic depression and mania
    B.   Neurologic disorders
        1.   Alzheimer's dementia
        2.   Epilepsy
        3.   Stroke (via release hallucination of seizures)
    C.   Complex multimodal peduncular hallucinations (thalamic infarction)
    D.   Metabolic derangements
        1.   Alcohol withdrawal
    E.   Drugs
        1.   Prescription: indomethacin, digoxin, bupropion, vincristine, cyclosporine, lithium, lidocaine, dopamine, topical homatropine, scopolamine, atropine, withdrawal of baclofen
        2.   Hallucinogens: marijuana, PCP, psilocybin, mescaline, LSD, 3,4-methylene-dioxymethamphetamine (Ecstasy), nutmeg
    F.   Release hallucinations (Charles Bonnet syndrome)
    G.   Visual migraines
II.   Palinopsia
    A.   Cerebral lesions
        1.   Right parieto-occipital area
        2.   Bilateral and left-sided lesions have been reported
        3.   Temporal and medial occipital lobe lesions
    B.   Drugs
        1.   Mescaline—occasionally permanent
        2.   LSD—occasionally permanent
        3.   3,4-methylenedioxymethamphetamine (Ecstasy)—occasionally permanent
        4.   Clomiphene
        5.   Trazodone
        6.   Interleukin-2
        7.   Nafazodone
    C.   Metabolic disorders
        1.   Nonketotic hyperglycemia
    D.   Psychiatric disorders
        1.   Creutzfeldt-Jakob disease
III.   Cerebral polyopia
    A.   Dominant or nondominant parietal or parieto-occipital lesion
    B.   Occipital lobe injury
    C.   Encephalitis
    D.   Seizure
    E.   Multiple sclerosis
    F.   Migraine
    G.   Tumor
IV.   Visual allesthesia
    A.   Wallenberg's lateral medullary syndrome
    B.   Lesion of the posterior parietal cortex
        1.   Infarction
        2.   Neoplasm
        3.   Trauma
        4.   Infection
        5.   Multiple sclerosis
        6.   Migraine (transient)
        7.   Seizure (transient)

        b.   Associative object agnosia—a generalized loss of object identification that often affects multiple categories of objects (eg, cars, animals, faces)

  C.   Visual-limbic disconnection

     1.   Definition: these syndromes develop due to disconnection of visual information from limbic structures involved in memory and emotions

     2.   Etiology: due to ventral occipitotemporal lesions that damage connections to limbic structures

     3.   Types:

         a.   Visual amnesia—modality-specific disorder in which patients are unable to learn new visual objects, patterns, and faces or to remember visual surroundings

         b.   Visual hypoemotionality—a rare syndrome in which emotional responses to visual stimuli are blunted or absent

IX. Visual hallucinations and illusions

  A.   Of the many etiologies of hallucinations and illusions (see Table 18-3), the following four categories are of the most importance to the ophthalmologist

     1.   Release hallucinations (Charles Bonnet syndrome)

         a.   Definition: hallucinations that frequently occur in patients who lose vision in both eyes regardless of the location of the causative lesion or lesions

         b.   May be simple (flashes of light, shapes) or complex (people, objects)

         c.   Patients are psychiatrically normal and usually not disturbed by the hallucinations

         d.   Occurs in 11% to 13% of blind patients

         e.   Worsens with social isolation

         f.   No clear treatment

     2.   Visual migraines (see Chapter 15)

     3.   Visual seizures

         a.   Occipital and less commonly temporal lobe seizures may cause unformed hallucinations similar to those experienced during a classic migraine attack

         b.   Temporal lobe and rarely occipital lobe seizures may cause formed visual hallucinations, mimicking Charles Bonnet syndrome

         c.   Distinguishing seizures from migraine is usually possible by careful history; however, seizure monitoring may be needed in some cases

         d.   Characteristics of visual seizures:

             i.   Usually lack the typical history of migraines

             ii.   Atypical frequency and duration of hallucinations

             iii.   Exhibit other seizure phenomena, such as eye deviation or rapid blinking

     4.   Visual perseveration

         a.   Definition: the pathologic persistence or recurrence of a previously seen visual image

         b.   Types:

i. Palinopsia
  a. Definition: the preservation in time of a previously viewed image
  b. Patients report seeing a previously viewed image immediately after it was seen or occasionally several minutes later
  c. Usually associated with an homonymous field defect and occurs in the affected portion of the field
  d. Etiology (see Table 18-3)
ii. Cerebral polyopia
  a. Definition: the preservation in space of an image (ie, seeing two or more images)
  b. Unlike diplopia, due to optic aberrations; images are equal in clarity
  c. Homonymous field defects are often present
  d. Etiology (see Table 18-3)

BIBLIOGRAPHY

Chapters

Burde RM, Savino PJ, Trobe JD. *Clinical Decisions in Neuro-Ophthalmology*. 3rd ed. St Louis, Mo: CV Mosby; 2002:114-135.

Lessel S. Higher disorders of visual function: negative phenomena. In: Glaser J, Smith J, eds. *Neuro-Ophthalmology*. Vol 8. St Louis, Mo: Mosby; 1975:3-4.

Rizzo M, Barton J. Central disorders of visual function. In: Miller NR, Newman, NJ, eds. *Walsh and Hoyt's Clinical Neuro-Ophthalmology*. 6th ed. Vol 1. Philadelphia, Pa: Lippincott Williams & Wilkins; 2005:575-645.

Articles

Barrett AM, Beversdorf DQ, Crucian GP, Heilman KM. Neglect after right hemisphere stroke: a smaller floodlight for distributed attention. *Neurology*. 1998;51:972-978.

Damasio AR, Damasio H. The anatomic basis of pure alexia. *Neurology*. 1983;33:1573-1583.

Damasio AR, Damasio H, Van Hoesen GW. Prosopagnosia: anatomic basis and behavioral mechanisms. *Neurology*. 1982;32:331-341.

Farah MJ. Agnosia. *Curr Opin Neurobiol*. 1992;2:162-164.

Girkin CA, Miller NR. Central disorders of vision in humans. *Surv Ophthalmol*. 2001;45:379-405.

Hausser CO, Robert F, Giard N. Balint's syndrome. *Can J Neurol Sci*. 1980;7:157-161.

Heywood CA, Gadotti A, Cowey A. Cortical area V4 and its role in the perception of color. *J Neurosci*. 1992;12:4056-4065.

Holroyd S, Rabins PV, Finkelstein D, et al. Visual hallucinations in patients with macular degeneration. *Am J Psychiatry*. 1992;149:1701-1706.

Jacobs L. Visual allesthesia. *Neurology*. 1980;30:1059-1063.

Manford M, Andermann F. Complex visual hallucinations. Clinical and neurobiological insights. *Brain*. 1998;121:1819-1840.

Menon GJ, Rahman I, Menon SJ, et al. Complex visual hallucinations in the visually impaired: the Charles Bonnet syndrome. *Surv Ophthalmol.* 2003;48:58-72.

Nobre AC, Sebestyen GN, Gitelman DR, et al. Functional localization of the system for visuospatial attention using positron emission tomography. *Brain.* 1997;120:515-533.

Schiller PH, Logothetis NK, Charles ER. Role of the color-opponent and broad-band channels in vision. *Vis Neurosci.* 1990;5:321-346.

Stoerig P, Cowey A. Blindsight in man and monkey. *Brain.* 1997;120:535-559.

Zeki S, Ffytche DH. The Riddoch syndrome: insights into the neurobiology of conscious vision. *Brain.* 1998;121:25-45.

Zeki S, Watson JD, Lueck CJ, et al. A direct demonstration of functional specialization in human visual cortex. *J Neurosci.* 1991;11:641-649.

Chapter 19

The Phakomatoses: Neurocutaneous Disorders

Angela R. Lewis, MD

I. **The phakomatoses defined**

   A. The phakomatoses are a group of disorders characterized by hamartomas of the skin, central nervous system (CNS), eye, and visceral organs

   B. Hamartomas are abnormal proliferations of mature cells normally found in the involved organ

II. **Neurofibromatosis type 1 (NF1)**

   A. Also known as von Recklinghausen's neurofibromatosis or peripheral neurofibromatosis

   B. NF1 occurs in approximately 1 in 3500 persons

   C. Decreased life expectancy. Mean age at death is 54.4 years

   D. Genetics
      1. NF1 may be inherited as an autosomal dominant trait; 30% to 40% of cases are due to spontaneous mutations
      2. The NF1 gene is located on chromosome 17 (17q12-22). The gene has 100% penetrance but is highly variable in its expression
      3. The NF1 gene, a tumor suppressor gene, produces a protein called neurofibromin, which negatively regulates the oncoprotein ras. Neurofibromin accelerates the conversion of active guanosine triphosphate (GTP) bound ras to its inactive guanosine diphosphate (GDP) form
      4. Mutations of the NF1 gene results in a loss of neurofibromin, which leads to an increase in cell growth and tumor formation

   E. Cutaneous lesions
      1. Café-au-lait spots are found in 99% of patients with NF1
         a. Flat hyperpigmented lesions
         b. Present at birth and increase in size and number with time
         c. Distributed randomly over the body but do not occur on the scalp, eyebrows, palms, or soles
         d. Histology: hyperpigmentation of the basal cell layer of the epithelium

2. Freckles are found in 81% of patients with NF1
   a. Hyperpigmentation of the groin, axilla, inframammary regions, and other intertriginous areas
   b. Usually present by age 6
3. Neurofibromas are benign tumors of the peripheral nerves
   a. Composed of axons, Schwann cells, and fibroblasts
   b. Localized (isolated) neurofibromas compose 80% to 90% of neurofibromas found in NF1
      i. Circumscribed lesion
      ii. Uncommon before age 6; will increase in size and number with age
   c. Plexiform neurofibromas compose 10% to 20% of neurofibromas in NF1
      i. Congenital
      ii. Extensive interdigitation into surrounding tissue
      iii. Associated with soft tissue hypertrophy
      iv. Rarely undergoes malignant transformation

F. Ocular lesions
   1. Lisch nodules
      a. Melanocytic hamartoma
      b. Tan, brown, or yellow domed-shaped lesions that protrude from the iris surface
      c. Uncommon prior to age 6, but increases in number with age
      d. Do not cause visual symptoms
   2. Eyelid
      a. Café-au-lait spots
      b. Neurofibromas—both isolated and plexiform. Plexiform neurofibromas of the upper eyelid are associated with defects of the sphenoid bone and with congenital glaucoma
   3. Orbit
      a. Orbital neurofibromas
      b. Defects in the sphenoid wing—may cause pulsating proptosis
   4. Optic nerve glioma (see Chapter 10)
      a. Predominant intracranial neoplasm in NF1. Occurs in 15% of patients with NF1
      b. Grade 1 pilocytic astrocytoma
      c. Occurs predominantly in young children; most optic nerve gliomas are diagnosed by age 6. Fifty to 75% are asymptomatic at time of diagnosis
      d. Fifty percent of patients with optic nerve and chiasmal gliomas will experience ophthalmologic problems: proptosis, strabismus, loss of visual acuity, papilledema
      e. Gliomas may involve the hypothalamus, leading to endocrine abnormalities (eg, precocious puberty, diabetes insipidus)

      f.   Magnetic resonance (MR) scanning essential in demonstrating optic nerve, chiasm, optic tract, and thalamic/basal ganglia/cerebellar involvement. Optic nerve and chiasmal gliomas are diagnosed by magnetic resonance imaging (MRI). On T_2 images, one sees a fusiform enlargement of the optic nerve

      g.   Few patients with symptomatic gliomas will require treatment, whether by surgery, radiation, or chemotherapy

      h.   Visual pathway gliomas may remain stable, enlarge, or regress (postbiopsy or spontaneously)

   5.   Corneal nerves may be enlarged in NF1

   6.   Retinal lesions are uncommon and nonspecific. Patients may have a combined hamartoma of the retina and retinal pigment epithelium (RPE) or an astrocytic hamartoma

G.   CNS lesions

   1.   Tumors of the CNS are common

      a.   Optic pathway glioma

      b.   Brainstem glioma

      c.   Schwannoma

      d.   Meningioma

   2.   Aqueductal stenosis

   3.   Macrocephaly

   4.   Headaches

   5.   Seizures

   6.   Impaired intellect

H.   Visceral lesions

   1.   Increased risk for malignancies

      a.   Neurofibrosarcoma

      b.   Malignant myeloid disorders

      c.   Rhabdomyosarcoma

      d.   Wilms' tumor

      e.   Pheochromocytoma

   2.   Skeletal abnormalities

      a.   Short stature

      b.   Pseudoarthrosis

      c.   Scoliosis

   3.   Hypertension may be secondary to a pheochromocytoma or renal artery stenosis

I.   Diagnostic criteria: must have at least two of the following to make a diagnosis of NF1

   1.   Six or more café-au-lait spots. Must measure at least 5 mm in prepubertal individuals and at least 15 mm in postpubertal individuals

   2.   Two or more neurofibromas of any type or one plexiform neurofibroma

   3.   Axillary or inguinal freckling

   4.   Optic nerve glioma

    5.   Two or more Lisch nodules

    6.   Distinctive osseous lesions, such as sphenoid dysplasia or cortical thinning

    7.   A first-degree relative with NF1 by the above criteria .

III. Neurofibromatosis type 2 (NF2)

  A. Also known as bilateral acoustic neurofibromatosis or central neurofibromatosis

  B. NF2 is seen in 1 in 40,000 persons

  C. Genetics

    1.   NF2 is inherited as an autosomal dominant trait

    2.   The NF2 gene is located on chromosome 22 (22q12). It is believed to be a tumor suppressor gene

    3.   The NF2 gene produces a protein called schwannomin or merlin, which stabilizes cellular membranes. It links cytoskeletal and extracellular proteins to the cell membrane

  D. Cutaneous lesions are uncommon. Rarely, patients will have a few (less than six) café-au-lait spots or peripheral neurofibromas

  E. Ocular lesions

    1.   Posterior subcapsular cataract

    2.   Epiretinal membrane

    3.   Combined hamartoma of the RPE and retina

    4.   Optic nerve sheath meningioma

  F. CNS lesions

    1.   Bilateral vestibular schwannomas are the hallmark of this syndrome

       a.   Typically present in the third decade of life

       b.   Symptoms include progressive hearing loss, tinnitus, and vertigo

       c.   Histology: schwannomas are benign tumors arising from Schwann cells

    2.   Schwannomas of other cranial nerves, and spinal and peripheral nerves

    3.   Meningiomas: optic nerve sheath, intracranial, intraspinal

    4.   Gliomas

    5.   Ependymomas

  G. Revised criteria for diagnosing NF2

    1.   Definite NF2: one of the following

       a.   Bilateral VIII nerve schwannomas

       b.   A first-degree relative with NF2 and a unilateral VIII nerve mass

       c.   A first-degree relative with NF2 and two of the following lesions: neurofibroma, meningioma, glioma, schwannoma, or a posterior subcapsular lenticular opacity

    2.   Presumptive or probable NF2

       a.   Unilateral VIII nerve mass and meningioma, glioma, schwannoma, or posterior subcapsular lenticular opacity

       b.   Multiple meningiomas and unilateral VIII nerve mass, glioma, schwannoma, or posterior subcapsular lenticular opacity

IV. Alternate forms of neurofibromatosis

A. Conditions showing some of the classic features of either condition (NF1 or NF2) but not in a typical manner

B. Alternate forms of NF1

    1. Segmental neurofibromatosis: patients have manifestations of NF1 limited to one or more areas of the body

    2. Familial café-au-lait spots: patients only have café-au-lait spots

    3. Familial spinal neurofibromatosis: patients have multiple neurofibromas along the spinal canal and café-au-lait spots

C. Schwannomatosis is an alternate form of NF2. The schwannomas are confined to the skin and spine. The VIII cranial nerves are spared

V. Tuberous sclerosis (TS)

A. Syndrome also known as Bourneville's disease

B. Incidence is estimated at 1:10,000 persons

C. Genetics

    1. TS is inherited as an autosomal dominant trait, but 66% of cases represent spontaneous mutations

    2. Two distinct genes can cause TS: TSC1 and TSC2

        a. The TSC1 gene is on chromosome 9 (9q34) and encodes a protein called hamartin

        b. The TSC2 gene is on chromosome 16 (16p13) and encodes the protein tuberin

        c. Inactivation of both alleles of either TSC1 or TSC2 is required to produce TS

D. Cutaneous lesions

    1. Adenoma sebaceum appears in 75% of patients with TS

        a. Reddish-brown papular rash in the malar region

        b. Histologically, these lesions are angiofibromas. They consist of vascular, fibrous, and dermal tissue elements

    2. Mountain-Ashleaf spots are seen in 90% of patients with TS

        a. Hypomelanotic macules

        b. Can be present at birth

        c. Best seen with ultraviolet light (Wood's lamp)

    3. Subungual/periungual fibromas are seen in 25% of TS patients

        a. Angiofibromas of the nail

        b. More common on toenails than fingernails

    4. Shagreen patches are seen in 20% of TS patients

        a. Connective tissue hamartoma

        b. Gross appearance: area of thickened skin, usually over the lumbosacral region

E. Ocular lesions

    1. Retinal astrocytic hamartoma

        a. Present in 75% of TS patients

        b. Multiple lesions are often found in one eye

          c.   Twenty-five percent of patients will have bilateral lesions

          d.   Rarely affects vision

          e.   Three types of astrocytic hamartoma

               i.   Type 1—flat, smooth, and semitranslucent

               ii.   Type 2—opaque, nodular, elevated, and calcified

               iii.   Type 3—combination of types 1 and 2

    2.   Patches of RPE depigmentation

    3.   Angiofibroma of the eyelids and conjunctiva

F.   CNS lesions

    1.   Cortical tubers (hamartomas)

          a.   Alterations in cerebral cortex pattern; affected gyri are enlarged and hardened

          b.   Disruptions in cerebral cortical cellular pattern leads to seizures and mental retardation. Size and number of tubers positively correlate with the level of cognitive impairment and severity of seizures in patients

    2.   Subependymal nodules

          a.   Irregular nodules that protrude into the ventricles from the subependymal layer and often calcify

          b.   Often enlarge and are then referred to as giant cell astrocytomas

          c.   May enlarge to cause obstructive hydrocephalus

G.   Visceral lesions

    1.   Lymphangiomyomatosis affects the lung parenchyma

          a.   Occurs in 1% to 6% of cases and only in women with TS

          b.   Can cause spontaneous pneumothorax and respiratory failure

          c.   Treatment includes hormonal therapy and lung transplantation

    2.   Renal system

          a.   Angiomyolipomas are composed of abnormal blood vessels, smooth muscle, and adipose tissue. These renal tumors are seen in 80% of patients with TS

          b.   Renal cysts are seen 15% to 20% of the time

          c.   Renal cell carcinoma occurs in 2% of patients

    3.   Rhabdomyomas of the heart are common, seen in 67% of patients

          a.   Rhabdomyomas are usually clinically silent

          b.   These lesions decrease in size and may disappear over time

    4.   Sclerosis of the calvarium and spine occur in 40% of TS patients

    5.   Pitting of tooth enamel is common

H.   Diagnostic criteria

•   Definite TS: either two major features or one major feature plus two minor features

•   Probable TS: one major feature plus one minor feature

•   Suspect TS: either one major feature or two minor features

    1.   Major features

          a.   Facial angiofibromas or forehead plaque

          b.   Nontraumatic ungual or periungual fibroma

          c.   Hypomelanotic macules (three or more)

      d.   Shagreen patch

      e.   Cortical tuber

      f.   Subependymal nodule

      g.   Subependymal giant cell astrocytoma

      h.   Multiple retinal nodular hamartomas

      i.   Cardiac rhabdomyoma

      j.   Lymphangiomyomatosis

      k.   Renal angiomyolipoma

  2.   Minor features

      a.   Multiple randomly distributed pits in dental enamel

      b.   Hamartomatous rectal polyps

      c.   Bone cysts

      d.   Cerebral white matter radial migration lines

      e.   Gingival fibromas

      f.   Nonrenal hamartoma

      g.   Retinal achromic patch

      h.   "Confetti" skin lesions

      i.   Multiple renal cysts

VI. Von Hippel-Lindau disease (VHL)

A.   Also known as angiomatosis of the retina and cerebellum

B.   VHL neoplasms are hypervascular and overproduce angiogenic peptides such as vascular endothelial growth factor

C.   VHL occurs in 1 in 36,000 persons

D.   Genetics

  1.   VHL is inherited as an autosomal dominant trait with incomplete penetrance

  2.   The VHL gene is on chromosome 3 (3p25-26). It is a tumor suppressor gene

E.   There are no cutaneous lesions

F.   Ocular lesion—retinal hemangioblastoma

  1.   Usually the first manifestation of VHL; can be missed in its early stages due to peripheral location and small size

  2.   Stages of a retinal hemangioblastoma

      a.   Stage 1—preclassical: lesion is small and without feeder vessels

      b.   Stage 2—classical: lesion takes on a globular shape and feeder vessels are evident

      c.   Stage 3—marked by extravasation of lipid and plasma

      d.   Stage 4—reached if a retinal detachment occurs

      e.   Stage 5—marked by blindness secondary to retinal detachment, glaucoma, or persistent uveitis

  3.   Fifty percent of patients will have bilateral eye disease. Sixty percent will have multiple lesions in one eye. Fifty percent will have severe visual loss

  4.   Histologically, hemangioblastomas are composed of capillaries and glial cells

  5.   This lesion can be treated with photocoagulation or cryotherapy

G. CNS lesions

    1. Hemangioblastoma

        a. Most often located in the cerebellum (52%), but can occur in the spinal cord (44%) and brainstem (18%)

        b. Usually asymptomatic until the third decade of life. Patients present with signs of raised intracranial pressure—headache, nausea, papilledema, and VI nerve paresis. May also have vertigo, nystagmus, and ataxia

    2. Syrinx

        a. May be located in the spinal cord or brainstem

        b. Symptoms include weakness and atrophy of the hands and arms, pain, and nystagmus

    3. Endolymphatic sac tumors

        a. Have been found to have the same genetic defects as other VHL tumors

        b. Patients present with hearing loss, tinnitus, vertigo, and facial weakness

H. Visceral lesions

    1. Renal cell carcinoma

    2. Pheochromocytoma

    3. Benign cysts of the kidneys, pancreas, liver, and epididymis

    4. Polycythemia: the CNS hemangioblastoma produces erythropoietin

I. Diagnostic criteria: patients must have one manifestation of the syndrome and a family member with a CNS hemangioblastoma

VII. Sturge-Weber syndrome (SWS)

A. Also known as encephalotrigeminal angiomatosis

B. Rare syndrome. Estimated frequency of 1:50,000

C. Hereditary pattern is unknown. Patients with SWS have normal karyotypes

D. Facial lesion—facial angioma

    1. This lesion is also referred to as a port-wine stain or a nevus flammeus

    2. Present at birth

    3. The reddish-purple lesion is usually unilateral and follows cutaneous distribution of V^1 and V^2. V^3 is less often affected. One, two, or all three dermatomes may be involved simultaneously

    4. Facial angiomas can be bilateral. Some patients have extensive lesions that involve the trunk and limbs

    5. Port-wine stain is associated with hemihypertrophy of the face

E. Ocular lesions

    1. Glaucoma is seen in 60% of patients with SWS. Sixty percent of patients will develop glaucoma prior to age 2

        a. Glaucoma is usually ipsilateral to the facial angioma

        b. More common in patients with facial angiomas involving the upper eyelid

        c. Glaucoma is believed to be secondary to an anterior chamber angle anomaly and/or elevated episcleral venous pressure

        d.   Glaucoma difficult to control

   2.   Choroidal hemangioma

        a.   Seen in 40% of patients with SWS

        b.   Ipsilateral to the facial angioma

        c.   Two types

            i.   Diffuse choroidal angioma is the most common—"tomato ketch-up fundus"

           ii.   Localized angiomas

        d.   Can cause hyperopia and retinal degeneration

   3.   Heterochromia iridis—the iris ipsilateral to the facial angioma may be deeply pigmented

   4.   Angiomas of the conjunctiva and sclera

F.   CNS lesion—leptomeningeal hemangioma

   1.   The angioma is located between the pia and arachnoid

   2.   Ipsilateral to the facial angioma; 15% of lesions are bilateral

   3.   Most often located over the parieto-occipital cortex

   4.   Underlying cortex is maldeveloped and hypoplastic

        a.   Cortical veins are absent or nonfunctional

        b.   Calcium deposited within the blood vessels and superficial layers of the cortex. Produces "tram-track" appearance on cranial computed tomography (CT) scanning

   5.   Consequences of cortical and meningeal lesions

        a.   Seventy-five percent will have contralateral seizures

        b.   Fifty-five to 85% of patients will have some form of learning disability

        c.   Hemiplegia

        d.   Homonymous visual field defect

G.   No visceral lesions

H.   Diagnostic criteria—patients must have two of these criteria

   1.   Facial angioma with ipsilateral intracranial hemangioma

   2.   Ipsilateral choroidal hemangioma

   3.   Congenital glaucoma

VIII. Wyburn-Mason's syndrome (WMS)

A.   Also known as retinocephalic vascular malformation

B.   Incidence and hereditary pattern unknown. Rare syndrome

C.   Cutaneous lesions rare. Some patients have a facial angioma

D.   Ocular lesions

   1.   Arteriovenous malformation (AVM) of the retina

        a.   This lesion is also known as a racemose angioma

        b.   It is unilateral and most often located in the posterior pole

        c.   Visual acuity can range from 20/20 to no light perception (NLP)

   2.   Orbital AVM

   3.   Optic nerve AVM

E.   CNS lesion—AVM of the CNS

1. Ipsilateral to the retinal AVM
2. Fifty percent will be symptomatic

F. Visceral lesions—patients may have AVMs of the ipsilateral maxilla, pterygoid fossa, mandible, and spine

G. Diagnostic criteria—the classic WMS consists of an intracranial AVM and separate retinal AVM

IX. **Ataxia-telangiectasia (A-T)**

A. Also known as Louis-Bar's syndrome

B. A-T occurs at a frequency of eight per million live births

C. Genetics
1. Inherited as an autosomal recessive trait
2. The A-T gene is on chromosome 11 (11q22-23)
3. The A-T gene encodes a protein called ATM, which is important for cell cycle control and DNA repair

D. Cutaneous lesion—telangiectasias of the skin
1. Occurs on exposed areas of skin—ears, nose, neck
2. Usually presents around age 4

E. Ocular lesions
1. Bilateral bulbar conjunctival telangiectasia
    a. Appears between the ages of 3 and 6
    b. Becomes more prominent with age
2. Ocular motility disturbances
    a. Patients first develop oculomotor apraxia
    b. Later, impairment of smooth pursuit
    c. Eventually, complete supranuclear ophthalmoplegia

F. CNS lesion—atrophy of the cerebellum
1. Atrophy particularly prominent in the cerebellar cortex and vermis
2. Clinical consequences of cerebellar atrophy
    a. Cerebellar ataxia becomes evident when the patient begins to walk; progressive; patients are wheelchair bound by age 10
    b. Dysarthria
    c. Chorea
    d. Dystonia
    e. Regression of intellectual milestones

G. Visceral lesions
1. Respiratory infections are frequent
    a. Hypoplastic thymus
    b. Hypoplasia of tonsils, adenoids, and lymphoid tissue
    c. Deficiency of IgG2, IgG4, IgA, and IgE
2. Patients with A-T have poor auto-DNA repair after exposure to ultraviolet light and radiation. This leads to a 100-fold increased cancer rate. They often develop leukemia and lymphoma
3. Elevated a-fetoprotein level

H.   Diagnostic criteria

1.   Characteristic neurologic features:

a.   Gait ataxia in the first 2 or 3 years of life

b.   Ocular motor signs and dysarthria by early school years. Subsequent movement disorders, worsening limb ataxia, facial hypomimia, swallowing incoordination, and peripheral neuropathy

2.   At least one of the following:

a.   Ocular telangiectasia

b.   Elevated serum a-fetoprotein level after 1 year of age

c.   Spontaneous or radiation-induced chromosomal breakage (colony survival DNA analysis)

X.   **Klippel-Trénaunay-Weber syndrome (KTWS)**

A.   KTWS is a sporadic disorder. Incidence and mode of inheritance is unknown

B.   KTWS is characterized by the following triad:

1.   Cutaneous capillary malformations

2.   Varicosities

3.   Bony and soft tissue hypertrophy

C.   Most common site is leg, followed by arm, trunk, and rarely head and neck

D.   Cutaneous lesion—port-wine stain

1.   Present at birth

2.   Found in 98% of patients with KTWS

3.   Darkens and thickens with age

E.   Ophthalmologic manifestations

1.   Port-wine stain of the face

2.   Orbital varix

3.   Heterochromia irides

4.   Varicosities of the retina

5.   Choroidal angioma

F.   CNS lesions uncommon

G.   Visceral lesions

1.   Varicose veins

a.   May be present at birth, but usually obvious during childhood

b.   Complications: lymphedema, stasis ulceration, pulmonary embolism

2.   Hypertrophy of bone and soft tissues

a.   Causes an increase in both length and girth of affected extremity

b.   Progressive during first several years of life

c.   Disproportionate enlargement of a single extremity can cause scoliosis and gait abnormalities

H.   Diagnostic criteria—patient must have two of these criteria

1.   Cutaneous vascular abnormality

2.   Soft tissue and/or bony hypertrophy

3.   Varicose veins

Bibliography

Chapters

Kerrison, JB. Phacomatoses. In: Miller NR, Newman NJ, eds. *Walsh and Hoyt's Clinical Neuro-Ophthalmology.* 6th ed. Vol 2. Baltimore, Md: Williams & Wilkins; 2005:1823-1898.

Shields JA, Shields CA. Systemic hamartomases. In: Manis MJ, Macsai MS, Huntley AC, eds. *Eye and Skin Disease.* Philadelphia, Pa: Lippincott-Raven; 1998:367-380.

Articles

Crino PB, Nathanson KL, Henske EP. Medical progress: the tuberous sclerosis complex. *N Engl J Med.* 2006;355:1345-1356.

Filling-Katz MR, Choyke PL, Oldfield E, et al. Central nervous system involvement in von Hippel-Lindau disease. *Neurology.* 1991;41:41-46.

Gihiczak GG, Meine JG, Schwartz RA, et al. Klippel-Trenaunay syndrome: a multisystem disorder possibly resulting from a pathogenic gene for vascular and tissue overgrowth. *Int J Dermatol.* 2006;45:883-890.

Jacob AG, Driscoll DJ, Shaughnessy WJ, et al. Klippel-Trénaunay syndrome: spectrum and management. *Mayo Clin Proc.* 1998;73:28-36.

Kaye LD, Rothner AD, Beauchamp GR, et al. Ocular findings associated with neurofibromatosis type II. *Ophthalmology.* 1999;99:1424-1429.

Lewis RF, Lederman HM, Crawford TO. Ocular motor abnormalities in ataxia-telangiectasia. *Ann Neurol.* 1999;46:287-295.

Patel U, Gupta SC. Wyburn-Mason syndrome: a case report and review of the literature. *Neuroradiology.* 1990;31:544-546.

Taylor AMR, Byrd PJ. Molecular pathology of ataxia telangiectasia. *J Clin Pathol.* 2005;58:1009-1015.

Theos A, Korf BR. Pathophysiology of neurofibromatosis type 1. *Ann Intern Med.* 2006;144:842-849.

Ward BA, Gutmann DH. Neurofibromatosis 1: from lab bench to clinic. *Journal of Pediatric Neurology.* 2005;32:221-228.

Weiner DM, Ewalt DH, Roach ES, Hensle TW. The tuberous sclerosis complex: a comprehensive review. *J Am Coll Surg.* 1998;187:548-561.

Yohay K. Neurofibromatosis types 1 and 2. *Neurology.* 2006;12:86-93.

Chapter 20

Ancillary Clinical Procedures

Patrick S. O'Connor, MD

I. **Superficial temporal artery biopsy**

   A.   The temporal artery is a terminal branch of the external carotid artery. Because of its ready accessibility and high frequency of involvement in giant cell arteritis, it is most often biopsied to establish the diagnosis

   B.   The artery lies in front of the ear over the zygomatic process of the temporal bone. It divides into a posterior parietal branch and anterior frontal branch (Figure 20-1A). The frontal branch lies above the temporalis fascia and follows a tortuous course across the forehead to an anastomosis with the supraorbital and supratrochlear branches of the ophthalmic artery

   C.   The frontal branch is usually chosen for biopsy. The artery is classically described as being nodular and tender when involved. However, the vessel may feel and look normal, yet prove abnormal on histologic examination

   D.   After the frontal branch is identified, the area should be prepared by shaving the overlying skin

   E.   The shaved area is scrubbed with Betadine (Purdue Pharma, Stamford, Conn) solution for 5 minutes with 4 x 4's. The area is then dried and a sterile plastic eye drape is applied to the biopsy area

   F.   The vessel is carefully palpated and its course marked for 4 to 5 cm

   G.   Plain 2% xylocaine is used for local infiltration. Epinephrine should be avoided because of its vasospastic potential. Five to 10 cc should be injected 1 cm to either side of the artery and parallel to, but not directly over, the artery itself

   H.   The skin incision is made with a No. 15 Bard-Parker blade (BD, Franklin Lakes, NJ) directly along the skin mark. Traction at each end of the incision site is used when making the full-thickness incision through the skin. 4 x 4's can then be used at the incision edges to control bleeding. Rarely is cautery or ligature needed

   I.   Subcutaneous blunt dissection is done using a hemostat or small blunt-nosed scissors. Dissection with sharp instruments is never performed. The frontal branch is identified above the temporalis fascia (Figure 20-1B)

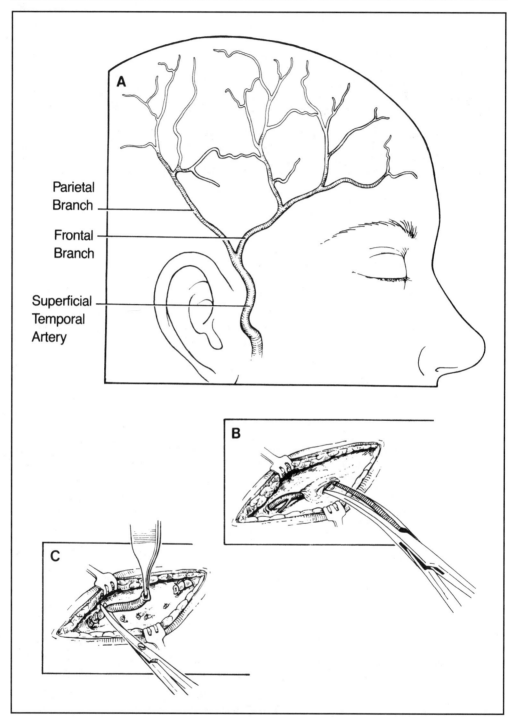

Figure 20-1. Steps in performing a superficial temporal artery biopsy. A. Localization. B. Blunt dissection. C. Removal of biopsy specimen.

J. If pulsations were obtained at the beginning of the procedure, the dissection bed is repeatedly palpated to identify the course of the artery

K. If the pulse disappears, several drops of proparacaine can be instilled on the wound, reducing vasospasm

L. Two 4-0 black silk sutures are passed below the artery, one proximally and one distally to permit manipulation without the use of instruments that could cause crush artifact. At least 3 cm of artery should be isolated and freed from surrounding tissue. Branches of the artery are ligated with 4-0 chromic sutures. The artery is ligated as far proximally and distally as possible. Three square knots should be placed with the silk sutures and the ends not cut too closely. Some prefer a double ligature proximally and distally (Figure 20-1C)

M. Once bleeding is controlled, the wound is closed with 6-0 nylon sutures. A pressure dressing is applied for 24 hours

N. The most common late complication is hemorrhage. There is one case report of a patient with asymptomatic internal carotid occlusion who suffered a stroke during biopsy of the ipsilateral temporal artery because of interruption of collateral flow. It may be prudent to compress the vessel for several minutes to ensure that critical collateral flow will not be compromised if it is removed

O. Skin sutures are removed in 5 days

II. **The Tensilon test**

A. Tensilon (edrophonium hydrochloride) is supplied in a single dose, 10 mg/1 mL breakneck vial

B. A definite endpoint must be selected. If the patient has no findings at the time of examination, testing should be postponed. If ptosis is present, it should be documented photographically before and after injection

C. If diplopia is present careful measurement of the deviation should be carried out before, immediately after, and 3 to 4 minutes following injection. Three types of responses may occur in myasthenic patients. Type 1 responses occur only in myasthenics while type 2 and 3 responses may be seen in nonmyasthenic ophthalmoplegia:

1. An improvement in alignment (large tropia becomes smaller)
2. A worsening of alignment (a small tropia becomes a large tropia)
3. A reversal of alignment (a left hypertropia becomes a right hypertropia)

D. Procedure in adults:

1. Tensilon should be drawn up in a 1 cc tuberculin syringe
2. 0.4 mg of injectable atropine should also be drawn up in another 1 cc tuberculin syringe
3. A 10 cc syringe is filled with injectable saline
4. A scalp vein needle is placed in a dorsal arm or hand vein
5. 1 mL of saline solution is injected and the patient observed for 1 minute
6. 0.2 mL of Tensilon is injected and the tubing flushed with 1 mL of saline, then observed for 1 minute
7. If no response, a bolus of 0.8 mL of Tensilon is injected and the tubing flushed with another 1 mL of saline; atropine is then connected to the tubing

8.   Atropine (0.4 mg intramuscularly) may be used to pretreat all patients 15 minutes before Tensilon testing, or used intravenously only to avoid undesirable cholinergic side effects (eg, bradycardia, angina, bronchospasm)

E.   In children and uncooperative adults, 0.4 mg of atropine is given intramuscularly 15 minutes prior to the injection of neostigmine (Prostigmin [Valeant Pharmaceuticals International, Aliso Viejo, Calif]) and the dose calculated as follows: weight (kg)/70 (kg) times 1.5 mg=dose. Patient is reexamined 30 to 45 minutes after injection

III.   Forced duction testing (Figure 20-2)

A.   In patients with acquired diplopia and an incomitant deviation, forced duction testing can eliminate the need for extensive neurologic investigation if restriction is found. Remember, many patients with thyroid myopathy have only subtle or no other signs of classic thyroid eye disease

B.   Three drops of topical proparacaine solution are instilled in the inferior cul-de-sac of each eye. During this time, a cotton-tipped applicator is soaked with similar solution

C.   The patient is asked to look in the direction of gaze limitation. The cotton-tipped applicator is placed on the conjunctiva anterior to the presumed restricted muscle

D.   The conjunctiva is grasped with toothed forceps and the globe passively rotated in the direction of the limited duction

E.   The same procedure is carried out in the fellow eye and the relative limitation compared. In subtle cases, repeated comparisons between the two eyes may be necessary

F.   At times with attempted forced ductions, the globe is displaced backward into the orbit. This phenomenon must be observed, or the examiner may believe the eye moves more easily than it actually does

G.   Occasionally, patients are not able to cooperate for forced duction testing. In these cases, measurement of the intraocular pressure in the primary position and again with the eyes moved into the direction of limited gaze is compared. A pressure rise of greater than 4 mm in moving from one gaze position to another is felt to be diagnostic of a restrictive process

IV.   Confrontation visual fields

A.   Many significant neurologic field defects can be found with simple confrontation techniques

B.   The best technique of finger-counting fields evaluates both sides of the vertical meridian with care taken not to move the fingers in various quadrants since many patients with a damaged occipital lobe can still appreciate motion in the blind field (Riddoch phenomenon)

C.   Procedure (Figure 20-3):

1.   One eye of the patient is occluded

2.   The patient is then asked to look at the examiner's nose while maintaining steady fixation. The test distance should be approximately 1 meter between patient and examiner

3.   Finger counting is then carried out in the four quadrants: superior temporal, inferior temporal, inferior nasal, and superior nasal. Between one and five fingers is presented and the number varied. The fingers are presented in a static fashion 20 degrees and 30 degrees from fixation

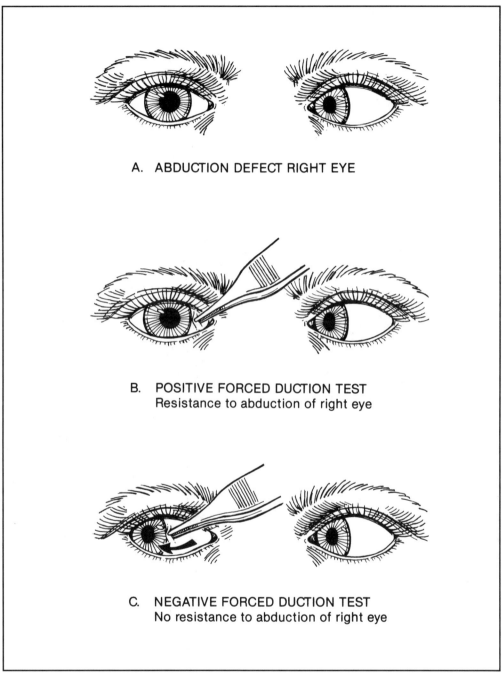

A. ABDUCTION DEFECT RIGHT EYE

B. POSITIVE FORCED DUCTION TEST
Resistance to abduction of right eye

C. NEGATIVE FORCED DUCTION TEST
No resistance to abduction of right eye

Figure 20-2. Forced duction testing.

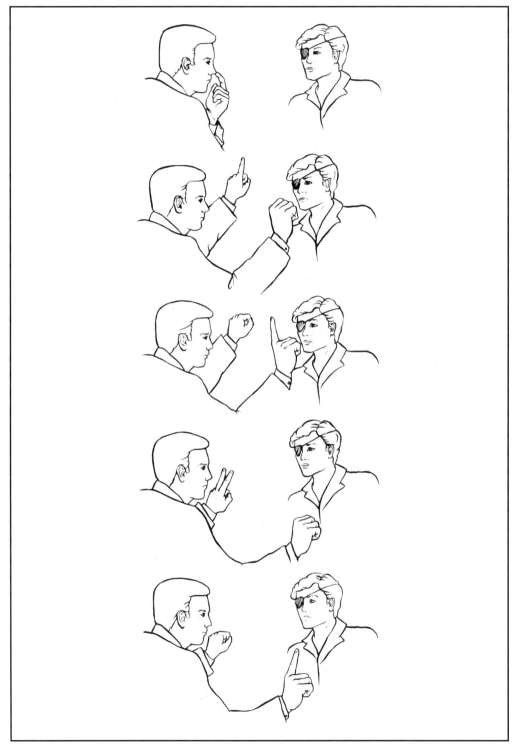

Figure 20-3. Confrontation visual field technique.

4. Double simultaneous stimulation (Oppenheim's test). The same number of fingers are simultaneously presented on each side of the vertical meridian with careful monitoring of the patient's fixation. Parietal lobe lesions can result in visual field inattention to simultaneous targets even when individually presented targets can be identified

5. Hemifield comparison. Again with controlled fixation, both hands are held on either side of the vertical meridian and the patient is asked to compare their appearance (ie, one "clearer" or "darker" than the other). The patient is always asked to point to the abnormal hand to reduce confusion. If, for example, the hand in the patient's temporal field appears dimmer, then both hands are again presented in the temporal field above and below the horizontal, and the patient is asked to identify the clearer of the two, allowing definition of whether the defect is denser above or below

6. The same procedure is carried out in the other eye

D. Finger-counting fields should be performed as part of every routine examination not just in patients suspected of having neurologic disease

E. A great deal of information can also be gained from subjective visual fields in which the patient covers one eye and focuses on the center of the examiner's face, usually the nose. The patient is then asked if he or she can see both ears simultaneously, the head, the chin, the examiner's shoulder, tie, etc. Frequently, scotomas not easily identified on perimetry are recognized as a central dimming by the patient when viewing the examiner's face. The same is also true for early inferior altitudinal defects that may be subtle on perimetry but easily identified by the patient on subjective examination

V. Optic nerve sheath decompression (Figure 20-4)

A. The orbital optic nerve can be approached surgically either medially or laterally

B. The medial approach is preferred, since it is technically easier and quicker, and avoids removal of the lateral bony orbital wall

C. A speculum is used to open the lids, and a lateral canthotomy is performed

D. A medial conjunctival peritomy is made, the medial rectus muscle is isolated on a muscle hook, a double-armed 6-0 coated Vicryl suture (Ethicon J-570, Somerville, NJ) is passed though the muscle close to its insertion, and the muscle is disinserted from the globe

E. Another double-armed 6-0 Vicryl suture (J-556) is woven through the stump of the medial rectus insertion, and this suture is used to pull the eye into an abducted position (see Figure 20-4A)

F. Single-armed 5-0 Dacron sutures (Davis & Geck 2919-23, Manati, Puerto Rico) are passed through partial-thickness sclera in the superonasal and inferonasal quadrants (see Figure 20-4A)

G. The two Dacron sutures are pulled firmly to position the eye in full abduction (see Figure 20-4A)

H. A malleable orbital retractor is placed between the disinserted medial rectus muscle and the globe to expose the optic nerve immediately behind the globe

I. Cotton-tipped applicators and cottonoids are used to retract orbital fat

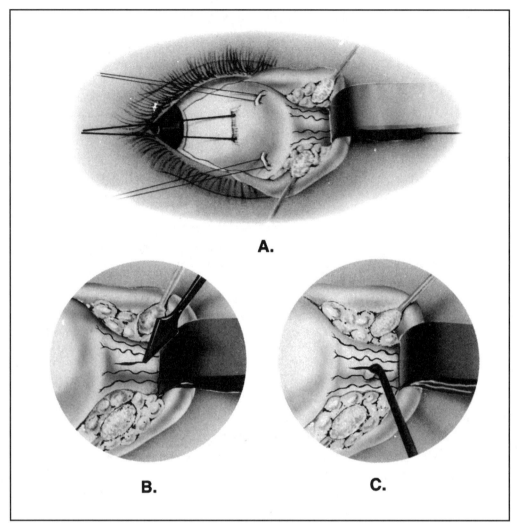

Figure 20-4. Medial approach for optic nerve sheath decompression (see text for details).

J.   The intrascleral course of the long posterior ciliary artery leads directly to the optic nerve

K.   Once exposed, an avascular segment of the nerve sheath is selected for fenestration

L.   Incision of the sheath is made with a sharp blade (MVR Untitome 5560, Beaver Surgical, Waltham, Mass) and extended approximately 5 mm (Figure 20-4B)

M.   A gush of cerebrospinal fluid is often seen with the initial incision

N.   Adhesions between the meninges and optic nerve are broken by passing a tenotomy or nerve hook into the fenestration (Figure 20-4C)

O.   Two to four fenestrations are made routinely, with lysis of the underlying adhesions

P.   Meticulous attention to hemostasis is required

Q.   The traction sutures are removed and the medial rectus is reattached at its original insertion

R.   The medial conjunctival incision is closed with an absorbable suture

BIBLIOGRAPHY

Chapters

Anderson DR. *Perimetry: With and Without Automation.* 2nd ed. St Louis, Mo: CV Mosby; 1987:228-249.

Burde RM, Savino PJ, Trobe JD. *Clinical Decisions in Neuro-Ophthalmology.* 3rd ed. St Louis, Mo: CV Mosby; 2002:177-178.

Articles

Chandrasekaran S, McCluskey P, Minassian D, et al. Visual outcomes for optic nerve sheath fenestration in pseudotumor cerebri and related conditions. *Clin Experiment Ophthalmol.* 2006;34:661-665.

Plotnik JL, Kosmorsky GS. Operative complications of optic nerve sheath decompression. *Ophthalmology.* 1993;100:683-690.

Sergott RC. Optic nerve sheath decompression. *Int Ophthalmol Clin.* 1991;31:71-81.

Shahinfar S, Johnson LN, Madsen RW. Confrontation visual field loss as a function of decibel sensitivity loss on automatic static perimetry. *Ophthalmology.* 1995;102:872-877.

Trobe JD, Acosta PC, Krischer JP, et al. Confrontation visual field techniques in the detection of anterior visual pathway lesions. *Ann Neurol.* 1981;10:28-34.

Tse DT, Nerad JA, Anderson RL, et al. Optic nerve sheath fenestration in pseudotumor cerebri. *Arch Ophthalmol.* 1988;106:1458-1462.

INDEX